A compilation of
nutritional wisdom by
Amy Bondar

optimum wellness through
sound nutrition

Published by Amy Bondar
Calgary, Alberta, Canada

Published by Amy Bondar
102 112 23 Avenue SW
Calgary, Alberta T2S 0J1

Library and Archives Canada Cataloguing in Publication

Bondar, Amy, 1976–

    Journey to optimum wellness through sound nutrition :
a compilation of nutritional wisdom / by Amy Bondar.
Includes bibliographical references.
ISBN 0-9781005-0-6
1. Nutrition. I. Title. II. Title: Sound nutrition.
RA784.B64 2006   613.2   C2006-903027-8

Disclaimer: The content of this book is based on the
knowledge and professional opinion of Amy Bondar,
unless otherwise cited. The information is not intended
to replace a one-on-one relationship with a qualified
Nutritional Consulting Practitioner (NCP) or wellness
professional nor is it intended as medical advice. The
nutrition tips are intended as a sharing of knowledge and
information from the research and experience of Amy
Bondar, NCP.

Page design and typesetting by Mazaa Design.
Printed and bound in Canada by Friesens.

eco-audit
By choosing 10% Post Consumer Recycled fiber instead
of virgin paper for the printing of this book, the following
savings to our natural resources were realized: trees
saved 1.14; wood reduced 657.98 lbs; water reduced
967.46 Gallons; landfill 102.59 lbs; net greenhouse
emissions 199.02 lbs; energy 1.59 BTu (000)

"I must say that each and every week, without fail, you provide an extremely relevant and informative tip. It is obvious that you put a lot of work into these and truly live what you teach and love to share with others." –Sherri Harty, Yoga Studio Manager

"I think you have a very professional approach to what you write and include in your articles and I look forward to each and every one." –Camelia Doyle, Pettibon Spinal Technician

"These are the foundational tools that allow you to live the life you want to live." –Jodi Ouellette, Lawyer

"I find these tips give me new ideas to work with, a lift when I'm struggling to put the time and effort into eating properly, and occasionally that pat on the back that keeps me coming back to making nutrition an important part of my life. Thank you!" –Laurie Legge

"It is not merely a 'tip of the week'—it is much more than that. I feel honored that you provide such a resource for clients. That is service." –Janice McTighe

"I have never before received such valuable information from anyone. Amy is well educated and knows how to put information forward to people on a level that they can understand. She truly wants to help each and every one of us, she inspires us and does all this without asking for anything in return. Amy has helped me out tremendously with setting my goals, reaching them and maintaining them. For that, I thank her from the bottom of my heart." –Carla Boland

"I love reading your e-tips week after week. They are very inspiring with wonderful information, creativity and of course knowledge." –Annabelle Bondar, author of *Messages from the Heart: Learning to Love Cancer*

To Mother Nature—
the source who nourishes us all

and

To all those who value health—
may the power of foods be the
greatest vehicle that guides
and supports you on your
journey to optimum wellness.

contents

❯with love and gratitude

This book is a manifestation of the inspiration I have received from two of my greatest mentors—Dr. Bruce Hoffman and Dr. John F. Demartini. You both have taught me that possibilities are endless and to believe in myself and in the power of my own dreams.

bruce

Four years ago—within one hour of fate closing the door on a direction my life could have taken—you stepped in and opened a different door. For that I am truly grateful. To work along with you, dedicated healer and grand visionary, day after day is a gift. You are my teacher and my friend. The first day I met you, you said, "If you stick with me you will be the most sought-after nutritionist in North America." I'm sticking with you, Bruce, because there is simply no better place. You set the bar high, and I am grateful— because your encouragement makes me want to be my best. Had I not worked with you, my world would be smaller, my knowledge and love for nutritional healing might have stagnated, and I would not have encountered the work of Dr. John Demartini, another master healer and teacher for our time.

john

Thank you for opening my heart, expanding my mind and awakening the spirit within me that I always knew but never knew how to manifest. You have taught me so much and my life has been transformed and enriched because of it. The greatest truth I have learned from you is that "we are surrounded by such magnificence that there is no way of handling it without tears of gratitude." I thank you for your own magnificence, for waking me up to mine, and inspiring me to open my eyes and heart to the perfection that surrounds me every day. It is a privilege to be one of your students.

sona

Thank you for always believing in me. Thank you for awakening my work with your gift of creative design. It means so much to me that you chose the tree of life as a symbol for my work and me. I am honored to have your love and energy bring my book to life. You are a beautiful friend and I am so grateful for the light, wisdom and creation you bring to my life.

kathy

Thank you for your time, honesty, interest and care in editing this book as well as opening my mind up to the possibilities of where it can go. Your suggestions and ideas enhanced my thoughts and writings and truly made the words dance on these pages.

kim

Thank you for your technical eye in the editing of this book. If I ever need help finding a needle in a haystack you are the woman I want on my team! Your precision, perfection and attention to detail is greatly appreciated and admired.

family

Dr. Demartini says, "Encourage your children's dreams... Have certainty in your children and see what happens." So let's see what happened... a successful practice, a book, and living the life I desire. And in between the encouragement and certainty I thank you for always supporting and challenging me along the way, because my growth has been dependant on both. There is a long history of successful businesses and private practices within both sides of our family and I am proud to be a part of that lineage. I believe it says a great deal about who we are and the passion within each of us to actualize our dreams.

clients

To all those who read my e-tips week after week, I thank you so much for the encouragement to continue to write, and for your wonderful feedback and support. This is your journey as much as it is mine and I look forward to continuing to support you as you support me on our path of learning, growing and mastering nutrition for optimal life!

To all of you I love… thank you for enriching my life.

With love, wisdom and gratitude,
amy bondar

The tree of life is a universal motif found in almost every ancient culture: a symbol of the uniting of heaven and earth, spiritual nourishment, knowledge, growth and enlightenment.

The tree is a powerful symbol of expansion towards the infinite and immersion in the finite. Its branches reach for the sun, soaking in the ever-present light, and its roots spread wider and deeper into rich, fertile earth. It is the link between heaven and earth, the unmanifest and the manifest. The tree becomes the intersection of spirit and matter from which one's potential to create is born. This ultimate symbol of life grows in every direction, both towards light and darkness and encapsulates both the feminine energy of sustenance and the masculine energy of growth, thus achieving a perfect balance in its embracing of the opposites.

With love, light and solid ground, a tree will grow forever and bear the apple of knowledge for all who seek it. Living in harmony with the source of life, eating the "fruits" of nature and always growing, learning and seeking more light while staying rooted in sound scientific research makes the tree of life the perfect symbol for one's nutritional journey.

While I was designing Amy's identity, I was struck by her fierce dedication to finding truth and wisdom in all facets of her life. I felt that this was a defining characteristic of Amy's personality and of her practice. I simply couldn't think of a more fitting symbol for Amy than the tree of life given its symbolic overtones of spiritual growth, wisdom and giver of life. And no matter how hard I tried to veer away from this image, I remained captivated by its multi-layered meaning. Over the years I've known Amy, I've seen her turn to nature to better understand her life and herself. A walk in the "enchanted forest" or time in the mountains often brings her new revelations. And as an impassioned Nutritional Consulting

Practitioner, Amy continues to seek new knowledge and integrate cutting-edge scientific research into her practice while remaining grounded in the wisdom of the ages. Her work invariably bears many fruits for her clients, just as it does for her.

>foreword by dr. bruce hoffman

At a recent conference, I was chatting with some of my colleagues who practise integrative medicine about what therapies make the most profound difference in patient outcomes. The one intervention unanimously agreed upon was nutrition—the changes that we all see when individuals adjust their nutrition in accordance with their metabolic or mind-body types. There is no question that nutrition is a key factor in helping people achieve their health goals.

For years now, the North American diet industry has focused on examining the calorie content of foods and nitpicking about whether the optimal diet is low fat, low carbohydrate, no fat, high carbohydrate, low protein, high protein or other endless variations. Modern-day nutrition has failed to take into account the influence of an individual's particular mind-body constitution and metabolic type. Very few nutritionists look at the body's biochemical inadequacies or at how environmental toxins block our metabolic pathways. It is rare that they look at the influence of specific food groups on one's gene expression and tap into research about the modifiable influence of food on our inherited gene pool. How many nutritionists consider the effect of unresolved emotions and limited belief systems on an individual's spiritual path or calling, and whether this disconnection is affecting the client's eating habits and sense of well being?

Amy Bondar recognizes that you are a fascinating, complex human being; a composite of mind, body and soul embedded in multiple, interlocking influences. She recognizes your uniqueness and avoids boxing you into a generic one-size-fits-all-program. Through the practice of nutrition and her individualized counselling techniques, Amy ensures that you are living at your maximal potential.

In this book, Amy touches on The 7 Levels of Healing™, an integral model of health care practiced at The Hoffman Centre for

Integrative Medicine. As an example, look at how Amy would begin to work with a client's nutritional program to optimize his/her health and well being.

At the first level—the level of the environmental influence on health—Amy asks about the client's exposure to environmental toxins and foods such as trans-fats, pro-inflammatory oils, high-fructose corn syrup, sucrose and sugar substitutes, such as aspartame. She educates her clients on how these toxic foods weaken one's physiology and begins a nutritional detoxification program that emphasizes whole foods.

At the second level, she analyses the physical body's structural and biochemical components, and the possible genetic influences that could play a role in disease outcomes. It is here that she determines the client's metabolic type and works with the client to determine any micro- and macronutrient deficiencies, food allergies or sensitivities. She also examines the client's exercise and stress-reduction routines. From this data Amy determines what lifestyle interventions are necessary and builds a customized nutrient-dense nutritional program.

At the third level—the level of physics and electromagnetism—Amy looks at the nervous system and the effect this has on digestion and the absorption of foods. She coaches clients on the importance of achieving a state of relaxation—a dominant parasympathetic state—before consuming meals. She describes how food traps light and it's this harvested energy that is absorbed when we consume colourful, live, fresh foods rather than dead food locked up in tin cans or frozen for eternity. This inherent life force found in whole foods is what enhances one's level of energy, sense of vitality and clarity. Here, Amy also speaks about the rhythms of nature and describes the classic four-season diet and how the body's needs change with the transitioning seasons.

At the fourth level—the level of unresolved emotional conflicts—Amy works to help the client with what is termed "emotional eating." She searches for underlying emotions that could be driving a person to unconsciously seek out food to fill emotional voids. This is also where a client recognizes the familial and social memories that influence his/her relationship to food.

At the same time, Amy begins to explore issues at the fifth level—the level of the ego and intellect. This is the home of our self-esteem and our internal dialogue—the voices inside which whisper to us an ongoing critique of who we are based on a composite of many voices and opinions projected onto us over a lifetime of exchanges and experiences. This is where the core issues about body image, self-worth and values stem from.

At the sixth level—the level of the personal soul, family and collective soul—Amy implements tools like Ayurveda to connect with the client's deepest unconscious influences. In Ayurvedic medicine, illness and disease are believed to take seat when we are disconnected from our true nature, which is termed Soul (Atman). When we are settled in the silence of our true selves, as observers of our minds, emotions and bodies, we are filled with a radiant bliss and joy that transcends the concerns of physical sensory-based reality. It is at this level that the choice maker is awakened, that part of ourselves that can consciously choose new behaviours to gain new outcomes. Amy will often suggest meditation as a tool to gain access to this deepest aspect of an individual's reality.

At the seventh level—the level of Spirit—Amy encourages her clients to see the larger context of their lives and makes sure that they carry with them a deeper sense of their life mission and purpose. It is at this level that Amy bridges nutrition with consciousness to see if a client is connected to their deepest spiritual path or calling. It is possible that a disconnection from this informing field may be why a client reaches into the refrigerator over and over again to fill a hole that is not physical in nature.

As you delve into the pages of this book, you will realize you are not engaging in the normal exchange between nutritionist and client. It's not about generic meal plans with simple advice about calories and carbs. In this book, you will awaken to the sheer joy of having a human body to take in the delights from nature's garden. You will find yourself in the company of a scholar, a healer and an inspired human being who draws on timeless traditions of healing.

With an open heart and enquiring mind, Amy will accompany you on your journey to knowing yourself in a whole new conscious way. In practicing Amy's sound nutritional wisdom, you will be inspired to live at your maximal potential in the body that you have grown to feed, nurture and love as the living treasure transporting you through this incredible experience of sentient life.

Food is one of the constants in our lives. We nourish from the moment of our conception, to the time we are born, right to the time of our physical death. We often eat five or six times a day, so what we eat must contribute to who we are, how we function and the level of energy at which we vibrate.

There is no question that every morsel of food we eat impacts the health of our bodies and every time we eat we have the power to influence our health. There is no greater nutritional truth than knowing with certainty that what we eat significantly affects our physical, mental, emotional and spiritual well being. Watching people tap into that truth and understand the relationship between the power of foods and the improvements in their own health is truly the greatest gift I receive from my work. It is why I continue to love what I do and do what I love—which is inspiring, educating and motivating people to realize the significant impact sound nutrition has on achieving optimum wellness.

Nutrition is both a science and a consciousness. Scientifically, it is about understanding how foods act and react to create health in the human body. Consciously, it is being awakened to the essence that fuels our mind, body and soul to fulfill our missions and purpose in life. For me, the marriage of scientific research and conscious nourishment is the foundation to actualizing wellness. I believe this is the nutritional paradigm we must embrace.

There is magnetic and electric power in foods. In my experience working at the Hoffman Centre for Integrative Medicine, 80% of symptoms disappear just by changing the diet alone. Most people I work with eat foods that work against their body type rather than for their body type, and so fail to nourish themselves when they eat. This is a recipe (pardon the pun) for perpetuating metabolic disease. As soon as we fuel the body according to type, great change begins to unfold. The truth is, the body knows how to heal itself, how to be healthy and how to function optimally—if given the right fuel. Sound nutrition is about understanding, knowing and learning to connect with your body so intuitively that you know with certainty what foods and ratios of these foods fulfill you to create balance and optimum wellness in your unique body. Sound nutrition is truly our greatest medicine. It is God-given, it is from the wisdom of Mother Nature and its power is transformational.

Twenty months ago, I began sending weekly "e-nutrition tips" to my clients as a way to stay connected with them. The truth is I love my clients. We are mutual partners in an optimum wellness journey, and each of us has a nutritional program that enlivens that journey. What I DIDN'T want for my clients was for their nutritional programs to become a temporary fix or a short-term trial or (groan) a diet. What I DID want for EVERY client was for him or her to wrap an invigorating, body, mind and soul-awakening, nutritional lifestyle into their personal way of being, healing and living. Indeed, this is food for following your dreams!

Still, one of the greatest feats of modern man and woman is maintaining focus on what we know will serve us. One of the greatest gifts we can give another is the inspiration to do just that. This was the purpose of my weekly "e-nutrition tips" and this is the gift I offer to you—nutrition tips that will inspire you and provide cutting edge insights and practical tools to use as you create and sustain your own bountiful, nourishing sound nutritional lifestyle.

The seventy-five tips in this book are a resource for all of you who value health and want to expand your knowledge and understand the true essence of sound nutrition. Throughout the book you may find references to the Hoffman Centre for Integrative Medicine. Though this is where I conduct my work, your nutritional success is not limited if you are not a personal client of mine or a patient at the Hoffman Centre. You can use this book as a guide, resource and source of inspiration, education and motivation while you fulfill your nutritional objectives with any wellness practitioner or on your own.

No rules come with this book. It can be picked up anytime, anywhere and used by anybody. Perhaps you are looking for a recipe or a new meal idea to create some variety. Maybe you are seeking power foods to enhance and optimize your nutritional lifestyle. You can refer to this book each season as a reminder of the most balancing foods to eat throughout the year. In times of struggle you can always find some motivating and inspiring words to keep you going. And if it is your soul that needs some nourishment you can be sure to find comfort inside these pages. Just look and you'll find nourishment for body, mind and spirit in this book. The tips are timeless and ageless and hold promise of comfort, inspiration and wisdom as you journey to optimum wellness through sound nutrition.

This book is not another fad diet, a how-to guide or another addition to the list of books that may leave you confused as a result of all the conflicting nutritional information that exists in our world.

This book is from the heart. It is about a truth so big that once you grasp it, feel it, taste it and live it, you will never again look at food in the same way. You will have transformed your life by nourishing yourself.

Yours in health,
Amy

The intention of this nutrition tip is to introduce the 7 Steps to Sound Nutrition™ program I created. So let's explore the 7 Steps so you can see and imagine the benefits to you, decide on your desired level of mastery, set your nutrition goals and plan your journey. Welcome to a grand adventure!

7 Steps to Sound Nutrition™ is possibly North America's most visionary, all-encompassing approach to nutrition. It combines scientific and holistic approaches, Eastern and Western insights. It provides you with your own customized nutritional road map and enables you to actualize and optimize your wellness goals.

This step-by-step program is intended to enhance your awareness of your own power and the power of nutrition in healing and living optimally. With each step, you unlock another secret code in the mystery of how foods react to and impact the health of your unique body type. You tap more fully into the real power of foods. You come to revel in the knowledge that every time you eat you choose how to influence your health—physically, mentally, emotionally and spiritually.

This comprehensive approach to nutrition will empower you to transform your life and become the master of your journey toward optimum wellness.

step one: your journey begins

The Comprehensive Nutritional Intake (CNI) I have designed looks at your entire body. You may see more questions about yourself and your lifestyle than any family physician has ever asked!

Its purpose is to build a knowledge bridge for both of us. The CNI helps you to understand who you are, and why your symptoms or conditions have manifested in the way they have. It enables you to begin to define your goals and teaches you to find purpose and meaning in creating a sound nutritional lifestyle by linking it to your highest values (see Tip 18). You begin to think about food in a new way and with a depth you might well never have experienced! The intake helps me understand your relationship with food and how your lifestyle dictates your current food choices.

At the end of our first meeting, I ask you to fill out an Advanced Nutri-Body® Analysis. This thorough questionnaire asks questions about your symptoms—how you feel physically, mentally and emotionally. Signs and symptoms are usually an indication that there are some nutritional deficiencies, excesses or weaknesses in the body that sometimes cannot be detected in blood or other laboratory tests. This in-depth analysis helps both of us listen to what your body is telling you, and to see just where your body is "at" nutritionally. Only then do we create your personalized road map. Your journey toward optimum wellness through sound nutrition has begun.

step two: building your nutritional foundation

The customized Nutritional Assessment and Recommendations I create for you based on Step One (and what you learn through these) form your foundation for wellness. Incorporating these recommendations into your wellness journey guarantees that you clean up your existing diet, correct nutrient deficiencies or excesses, ensure balanced macronutrient (proteins, essential fats, carbohydrates) ratios, strengthen the liver and digestive system, balance the endocrine system, alleviate symptoms and improve overall health conditions.

These recommendations offer longer-term value, too; they contain vital information both for preventative health and for slowing the aging process. This nutritional foundation is body, mind and soul-awakening, allowing you to use the power of foods to influence your biochemistry in a positive way. At Step Two, you truly

see that the slightest eliminations, additions and adjustments to
your diet can make a significant difference in how you feel!

step three: fueling your metabolic type

By now, your foundation has been established and you are moving
to a greater state of balance in the body. Now is when you and the
future of medicine join together. Your new catch phrase is "Metabolic Type." Quite simply, you'll want to determine and understand
you so that you can invite wellness in.

Metabolic typing is about fueling your autonomic nervous
system (ANS), which is the "grand regulator" of every metabolic
process in the body. When you understand how your unique ANS
functions, then you will know exactly which foods and what ratios of
macronutrients your body will need to produce enough energy to
function optimally according to your genetic code. When you balance the ANS, every cell, tissue, organ and system in the body will
work efficiently and when that happens, wellness sets in. In some
cases, disease can be reversed or prevented. Knowing your metabolic type takes the guesswork out—"What can I eat?"—so you can
progress on your journey to optimum wellness. It will give you certainty that the foods you are choosing are "just right" for your unique
biochemistry. When you have balanced your biochemistry you will
have long and lasting energy, your mental state will be sharp, emotions balanced and your weight will normalize. Your meals will also
always leave you feeling satisfied, satiated and free of cravings.
Knowing your metabolic type (one of carbohydrate type, mixed
type or protein type) is the key to your nutritional mastery.

step four: feeding your ayurvedic constitution

In Step Four, I work with you to create and redefine your lifestyle
for your individual body type (because ultimately at the Hoffman
Centre we want to guide and support you to adopt a healthier

lifestyle so you never again experience the health state with which you originally presented). Recognizing and feeding your Ayurvedic Constitution becomes the next essential step on your journey to optimal wellness.

Ayurveda means the science of life. It is one of the oldest healing systems that exist today. It is about helping you understand you—your personality type and your body type. Only when you know who you are and the elements that make you up can you consciously choose foods to keep those elements in balance.

For example, if you are a pitta (one of the three Ayurvedic body types or doshas), then you would know that you are made up of fire and water elements. Based on that understanding, you would learn that hot and spicy foods kick your fiery element way out of balance, while bitter foods cool and pacify the fire within. You would also learn, for instance, that Bikram yoga, saunas and noisy places over-stimulate your fiery element. You begin to understand which exercise or style of yoga is right for you, the best times for you to meditate, what imbalances your dosha, which spices are the best to use on your foods to create the right tastes at every meal, which massage oil and aromatherapy is most pacifying, and which herbal teas are most balancing for your unique constitution. Most importantly, Ayurveda is about creating and maintaining balance in the body because without balance, wellness cannot manifest.

step five: soulful nourishment

The first four steps are about what you eat, but this step moves into why you eat and how you eat. This step offers an incredible opportunity for breakthrough in nutrition and wellness, and is as important to your success as every prior step on the journey. Soulful nourishment presents as challenge and opportunity in many forms. This step, too, takes many different forms, whether it is overcoming emotional eating, using the Demartini Method® to collapse body image issues or other stressors in your life that are preventing you from eating well, learning how to eat consciously (see Tip 35), creating a sacred table (see Tip 71), using food to enhance and awaken your spirit, tapping into the meaning of food and how it has influenced your life (see Tip 68), or helping you overcome obstacles or "self-sabotage" moments that prevent you from carrying on with your nutritional lifestyle. Whatever your challenges are, they are all important pieces to consider on your journey. Eating is one thing, but nourishing yourself is another. It takes soulful nourishment to manifest true physical, mental, emotional and spiritual well being.

step six: seasonal eating

Connecting to the seasons and transitioning your food choices as the seasons change is an incredibly important tool for you to master. At this nutrition step you learn how to maintain balance throughout the year, how to prevent common cold and flu, how to listen to your body, how to be in tune with Mother Nature, how to connect to the earth and environment by eating what is seasonally available, how to create variety from season to season and the importance of adjusting your lifestyle as each season turns. There is a perfection and purpose to the foods we receive at each season and having awareness of that magnificence is an integral part of your nutritional journey. When you tap into that power and learn how to transition your diet seasonally, you will have gained knowledge in how to eat year after year. This is when you will truly have adopted sound nutrition as an infinite lifestyle.

step 7: evaluating your success

One of the high points of a journey is the time when you stop, look back and revel in just how far you have come. How do you measure progress on your journey to optimal wellness? You complete and compare your new Advanced Nutri-Body® Analysis with the one you completed when you started your journey. You will discover just how much you have corrected nutrient deficiencies, strengthened weak organ systems, revitalized your immune system and alleviated health concerns and conditions. At this moment you will know if you have actualized your health goals, created a new, balanced, healthier lifestyle and achieved your goal of optimum wellness. It is here that you can set a new path for yourself, new goals and travel with certainty on your infinite journey to wellness.

So there you have it, the 7 Steps to Sound Nutrition™. If you've been at Step Two for some time now, consider moving on to Step Three. If you have found your personal fuel mix with metabolic typing, then move to Ayurvedic nutrition and create a lifestyle that supports your dosha. If you continue to "self-sabotage" and struggle implementing the basic foundation, then it may be time to jump to Step Five. There is no right or wrong path on your wellness journey, and sometimes taking a step out of sequence will serve you well. Everybody's journey is unique. Just know that there is so much more than what is available to you in Steps One and Two. I urge you to continue to journey through each step to reach your nutrition goals and master your wellness potential.

Soy has been touted as a "super-food" for years, yet lately it has become one of the most hotly debated, controversial topics among researchers, health care practitioners and nutritionists.

There are many health benefits to eating fermented soy products such as miso, amakaze, natto, tamari and tempeh—all found in health food stores. These foods contain amino acids, B vitamins, vitamin E, vitamin K, phosphorus, calcium, iron and antioxidants (isoflavanoids). They promote the beneficial bacteria that keep the colon balanced and healthy. Fermented soy foods are safe, healthy and promoted because the long fermentation process deactivates antinutrients and cuts down otherwise high isoflavone levels. So if you like to supplement your diet with vegetable protein sources from time to time, enjoy these fermented soy foods, in moderation: 25–100 mg of fermented soy up to three times a week.

On the other hand, for optimum wellness avoid all processed soy foods such as soy burgers, soy nuts, bottled salad dressings, soy milk, soy cheese, soy protein bars, flavored tofu, soy ice cream, soy deli slices and soybean oil. "North-Americanized" soy foods are extremely dangerous. These foods are just as unhealthy as the other processed, manufactured foods found in most aisles of the grocery store (which are full of additives, preservatives, binders and fillers detrimental to health). Carcinogenic toxins, residues and petroleum have been found in factories that process soy. These foods lose much of their nutrient availability when processed, which is why many of them are fortified with nutrients. Don't be fooled by a label that lists soy ingredients. That doesn't mean it is healthy. Instead, flash a mental "danger" sign whenever you see processed, manufactured foods—including soy.

Some writers cite soy-based diets as a cause for lower incidences of breast cancer and other diseases among Asian populations.

But remember, a typical Asian diet, when compared with a typical Western diet, is higher in fruits, vegetables and essential fatty acids and void of fast-food, junk foods and processed foods! It is also important to note that in Asian cultures fermented soy is the norm. Fermented soy is nutritionally far superior to the danger-prone processed soy foods more common in North America. Consider also the quantities of soy consumed. In Taiwan, for example, most people eat very low quantities of soy, typically 36 grams a day. North Americans, on the other hand, are consuming increasingly larger quantities of the wrong kind of soy—the processed soy found in packaged, manufactured foods.

Beware of the quantity of soy you eat. Soy contains an antinutrient called a goitrogen, which blocks the production of the thyroid hormone, a hormone that plays an integral role in the regulation of metabolic activities. According to Dr. Kaayla Daniel, in *The Whole Soy Story,* "over 70 years of studies show that soy is a goitrogen and eating large quantities of soy greatly affects the thyroid."[1] In fact, there is a high correlation between soy consumption and hypothyroidism. Perhaps this is why we are seeing so many more thyroid disorders than ever before. If you have a weakened thyroid (hypothyroid) or any other thyroid disorder, soy foods should be completely eliminated from your diet.

Soybeans are very high in another antinutrient called phytates, which prevent the absorption of essential minerals such as calcium, magnesium, zinc and iron. A common hidden food allergy, soy has been known to weaken the immune system and hinder digestion. My strongest professional concern about all but small quantities of fermented soy is that soy can affect estrogen levels and alter a woman's menstrual cycle. As Dr. Joseph Mercola, a leading wellness expert, states, "two glasses of soy milk a day can drastically affect menstruation."[2]

So while some researchers say soy protects against breast and other hormone dependant cancers, others say soy accelerates the rate of breast cancer and does not have as much of a protective role as we were once led to believe. In other words, soy may be pre-ventative if consumed before cancer develops, but the role of soy consumption after cancer has developed is less clear. What is clear is that high amounts of soy should not be part of a cancer treatment plan, especially for women with estrogen-receptor positive breast cancer or women who are taking the drug tamoxifen citrate.

attention: men

Soy diminishes testosterone and libido. (It has been said that tofu was developed in monasteries to keep monks celibate!)

soy and babies

Soy infant formulas should not be given to babies because they contain extremely high amounts of manganese. In fact, accord-ing to Mercola, they contain eighty times more manganese than human breast milk or cow's milk, which is a toxic level for infants. An infant's liver, intestines and brain can neither handle nor eliminate this excessive amount. Dr. Daniel reports that excess manganese goes into the brain, alters biochemistry and causes free radical damage. Some research has linked Attention Deficit Disorder and violent behavior to this excessive amount of manganese. It takes six months for an infant's liver to fully function at full capacity. This means that infants cannot process high levels of heavy metals, such as the aluminum and fluoride found in infant soy formula.

Soy formula can also stunt the growth of infants by negatively affecting the thyroid. The level of soy estrogens in soy infant for-mula is startlingly high. According to the research done by Dr. Daniel, the blood of infants fed with soy formula contains 13,000–

22,000 times the amount of estrogen found in the blood of infants who are breast fed or organic-fed cow's milk. Daniel believes that we are over-estrogenizing our babies. For girls this means going through puberty, sprouting breasts, pubic hair, etc. at much earlier ages than ever before. For boys, Dr. Daniel correlates over-estrogenizing with late puberties, small penises, low sperm counts and the growing of breasts.

Studies are raising such concern in Europe that British and Swedish governments are taking a health stand against the use of soy infant formulas. Unfortunately, this is not the case in North America. In fact, a popular research paper often cited in the *Journal of the American Medical Association* that touts the safety of soy formula for infants was (we now know) funded by a soy company. Bottom line: never choose soy formula for newborn babies. Rice or goat milk-based formulas are preferable if breast-feeding or cow's milk is not an option.

It gets worse. Most soybeans are genetically modified; they contain one of the highest levels of pesticide contamination of all foods. Just recently I read that, to remove soy's natural toxins, soybeans go through acid washing in aluminum tanks, which results in leaching this toxic heavy metal into the final soy product.

The bottom line: If you are going to eat soy, eat it in moderation (up to three times a week). Eat only fermented soy products. Avoid all processed soy foods. Avoid soy entirely if you are pregnant, have hypothyroidism, or have been diagnosed with estrogen-receptor positive breast cancer. If you are a woman over forty or post-menopausal, and have never eaten soy, it is not wise to start now, at a time when hormones are drastically changing. Absolutely no infants should be on soy formula. If you are a vegetarian or vegan and are eating processed soy products, I highly recommend coming in for a nutritional assessment. Many wellness practitioners are seeing increasing numbers of vegetarians who are sick—and the more soy they eat, the sicker they become.

For all my clients and readers, err on the side of caution. Read the ingredients of every food you buy and avoid any foods with soybean oil, soy isolates, soy lecithin and so on. At this time there are far too many conflicting and startling research findings to promote soy as a "super" food.

If you are interested in more information on this hot topic, I highly recommend Daniel's *The Whole Soy Story.* It is highly informative, carefully researched, and a reputable, readable resource on soy.

home on the range

"The best part of dinner is not what you eat, but with whom you eat." –Unknown

Bison, also known as buffalo, is one of the healthiest and delicious red meats available today and is recommended as part of your optimum nutritional lifestyle. Low in saturated fat (5%) and cholesterol and high in protein, iron, zinc, vitamin B12 and essential fatty acids, buffalo is a nutritionally superior meat. In fact, according to the USDA handbook, one serving of bison meat provides 34% of the daily recommended amounts of protein, 32% of zinc, 33% of iron, 10% of niacin, 20% of phosphorus, 14% of Vitamin B6 and 42% of selenium.

Roasted bison has approximately:
- 60% more calcium,
- 500% more iron and
- 350% more zinc

than roasted skinless chicken breast.

Roasted bison has approximately:
- 200% more iron,
- 30% more zinc and
- 30% more potassium

than pan fried pork chops.

Roasted bison has approximately:
- 55% more calcium and
- 35% more iron

than round beefsteak.[1]

Bison truly are home on the range. They feed on grass alone. You won't find bison force-fed grains in feedlots. This makes bison a superb non-allergenic, easy-to-digest food source for those with gluten sensitivities or compromised digestion. Bison is free of all hormones and antibiotics typically found (in dangerously high quantities) in commercial beef.

Bison tastes great. It is very lean (leaner than a skinless chicken breast). It is tender and very quick and easy to cook. You can purchase bison ground, as patties, steaks, roasts, jerky, sausage and even pepperoni sticks (an excellent healthy snack for children and adults). You can find bison in the frozen foods section at any health food store. Farmer's markets carry it, as do specialty butcher shops.

Pick up some buffalo this week and try this fabulous recipe:

warm bison salad[2]

1 lb boneless sirloin bison steak
2 tbsp olive oil
½ tsp salt and pepper, each
1 ½ cups sliced red onion
2 cloves garlic minced
½ tsp dried rosemary
1 tbsp wine vinegar
2 tsp Dijon mustard
6 cups lightly packed torn fresh spinach

1   In a non-stick skillet, heat half of the oil over medium heat. Sprinkle both sides of steak with a pinch of salt and pepper. Cook steak for 4 minutes per side. Remove to plate and let stand for 5 minutes before slicing thinly across the grain.

2 Add onion, garlic, rosemary and remaining salt and pepper to pan. Cook over medium heat for 4 minutes, until onion is softened.

3 In a serving bowl, whisk together remaining oil, vinegar and mustard. Add onion mixture and spinach. Toss to coat. Arrange slices of bison steak over top. Serves 4.

Until next time, happy buffalo eating!

"We are indeed much more than what we eat, but what we eat
can nevertheless help us to be much more than what we are."
–Adelle Davis

When following your sound nutritional lifestyle you will experience
the true power of foods. You will find that the slightest eliminations,
additions and adjustments you make to your diet result in a significant difference in how you feel. The first thing you are likely to
notice is how your physical symptoms—your whole "symptomatology"—changes with the health of the body and mind improving
and toxicity symptoms diminishing (headaches, fatigue, mental
fog, acne, excess body fat and compromised digestion, to name
a few).

But the power of foods goes far beyond feeding the physical
body. What we eat significantly impacts how we see and what
we do. What we eat amplifies our understanding of who we are.
Many of the recommendations I make for your diet are designed
to improve more than your physical state. They are intended to
awaken your awareness of your own magnificence and help you
maximize your true potential.

powerful foods and powerless foods

Take a moment and think about your friends, colleagues or children who fuel themselves on sugared cereal, pop, fruit juice,
candies, chips, chocolate bars, junk food, processed, packaged,
factory-made food, endless cups of coffee, nutrient-deficient cafe-
teria food, canned or microwaved vegetables and so on. These are
dead foods. There is no energy or life force in them. People who
fuel themselves on these foods typically resonate the same way.
They have no energy, life force, magnetism, or spark. They com-
monly experience mental fog, lack of clarity and focus (sometimes

diagnosed as Attention Deficit Disorder) all signs that the mind is malnourished. They function below their capabilities and do not create all that they can or desire. These are people not living up to their true potential.

In contrast, those who fuel on fresh, vibrant, colorful, organic whole foods—foods that grow and subsist in nature—are "alive" because they are eating "live" foods. "Live" foods create energy, light, vibrancy and overall well being. In fact, according to Dr. Fritz Albert Popp, PhD, a leading physicist, when we eat live, whole foods, we are actually ingesting photons of light. Since a photon is a unit of radiant energy, we are ingesting both light and radiant energy! Popp has researched extensively the way in which vitamins, minerals and live foods (especially the chlorophyll found in dark leafy greens and wheatgrass) become the source of our energy; they are, in fact, carrier substances for light. Canned, microwaved and overcooked foods lose this light and energy.

Photon-rich foods are the foods that I promote and urge you to focus on in your nutritional lifestyle. Why? These are the foods that will take you to a higher state of wellness. I cannot emphasize this point enough. Connect with the power of these foods! Shop for them, eat them and appreciate them for more than just clearing up your physical symptoms. They are the means to create a fuller, richer, happier, more purposeful YOU! As they fill your being with light and energy, they help you be more and achieve more than you had thought possible.

Focusing on photon-rich foods makes grocery shopping a whole new adventure. When you shop at local health food stores and markets, you can feel the energy, light and vibrancy of foods. It is a difficult feeling to explain, but if you look, you'll recognize it. Because these foods have a live magnetic force, shopping for as well as eating them will feed your mind, body and spirit. You cannot feel the same energy when shopping at large industrial supermarkets, where food is treated like house wares. Amidst the endless aisles of manufactured dead foods in commercial grocery stores, the energetic resonance of live foods cannot be felt. The outer ring holds the energy, light and vibrancy, so stick to that and the next time you go for groceries, see if you can resonate with that same feeling I speak of.

As you journey to optimum wellness through sound nutrition, switch your food energy focus! Switch off focusing on foods to feed a physical hunger or an emotional desire. Switch on focusing on foods to maximize your energy, wellness and, ultimately, the power of you.

coffee—"that which excites and causes the spirits to rise"

Although coffee and coffee houses dot every urban landscape in North America, and new coffee drinks are slurped down as fast as they appear on the market, this trend is not new. Coffee houses date back to the ninth century. Drunk in long draughts, coffee was a delicacy, enjoyed among friends and a centerpiece of social and economic ritual. It was used therapeutically as a remedy and tonic. It was a source of income for many. For some, as illustrated below, it was used for inspiration.

In *History of Food,* Maguelonne Toussaint-Samat tells a legendary story about the effects of coffee on one religious leader.

> A few moments after tasting this mixture, his heart began beat-
> ing so fast that he had to lie down, but instead of falling asleep
> he felt extraordinarily lucid. His brain becoming active as in his
> youth was teeming with brilliant ideas. The Imam, a man of con-
> siderable intellectual powers, became even more knowing.[1]

Obviously coffee was and still is extremely potent—which is why it was only enjoyed or used from time to time. But like so much else in Western culture, coffee is consumed in excess (i.e. grandéed). Whether or not the indulgence has become addiction, excessive coffee consumption has become extremely detrimental to our health. It is a key contributor to many symptoms and conditions of imbalance, "dis-harmony" and "dis-ease." The following are just some of the dangers of excessive coffee consumption. Perhaps this will give you some insight into why I recommend eliminating frequent coffee consumption from your sound nutritional lifestyle.

- Coffee intensifies stress, causing an average 40% increase in adrenaline. This results in higher blood pressure, heart rate, perspiration, muscular tension, nervousness and irritability.
- Coffee increases the secretion of stomach acid by 400%, contributing to development of gastritis and peptic ulcer.
- Coffee is linked to ovarian, bladder and kidney cancer, doubling the risk of bladder cancer.
- Coffee drinkers have a 50% higher risk of heart attack than those who do not drink coffee.
- Coffee stimulates the pancreas and adrenal glands; it intensifies hypoglycemia and weakens the adrenal glands' ability to respond to stress.
- Coffee increases intellectual speed, not intellectual power (working faster but not smarter).
- Coffee is extremely dehydrating.
- Coffee increases the risk of miscarriage and can double the rate with just 163 mg a day—one cup!
- Coffee has an adverse effect on an unborn baby's muscular development and nutritional balance and increases the risk of birth defects.
- Coffee reduces fertility. More than one cup a day makes women half as likely to conceive.
- Coffee contains large amounts of polycyclic hydrocarbons (PAHs)—some of the most powerful of carcinogens (also found in charcoal-broiled meat).
- Coffee leaches many nutrients from the body, including magnesium, potassium, calcium, zinc and B vitamins, as well as inositol and biotin. It interferes with iron absorption. Women who drink one cup or more daily have significantly lower bone density after they reach menopause.

- Coffee is a major dietary source of cadmium, a heavy metal that is carcinogenic and immunosuppressive, and promotes prostate hypertrophy and cancer.
- 5000 mg of coffee has been known to be lethal to a 5-year-old child.
- Decaffeinated coffee contains methylene chloride, a toxic solvent that can affect the thyroid gland.
- Roasted coffee is a potent source of free radicals and of benzene, which contribute significantly to chronic disease and cancer.[2]

So, there you have it. If that doesn't make you want to stop the java jolt, read *America's Favorite Drug: Coffee and Your Health,* by Bonnie Edwards (the source of many of these statistics).

Instead of grabbing that cup of coffee first thing in the morning, stop to focus on the power of food to energize your body and awaken your mind. Switch from coffee to warm water with lemon first thing in the morning (this will stimulate your digestive enzymes and liver and get your bowels moving). Turn your coffee breaks at work into an herbal tea break or a glass of water followed by a quick brisk walk outside to re-energize your mind and spirit. Visit local teahouses for organic herbal teas. You can still go to Starbucks or your other haunts, but instead of grabbing coffee, treat yourself to an herbal tea.

If it is the coffee taste you want at times, try Teeccino—an herbal coffee alternative blended from herbs, grains, fruits and nuts that are roasted and brewed just like coffee, but without the undesirable effects of coffee. The ingredients include roasted carob, barley, chicory root, almonds, figs, dates and natural coffee flavor. You can find this product at most health food stores.

There is a continual ping-pong of benefits and drawbacks to drinking coffee among researchers and wellness practitioners.

Knowing that we may never find a definitive answer, the key is to tap into your unique body and ask, "Is it right for me?" This is where the ancient wisdom of Ayurveda and modern science of metabolic typing come into play. Typically vata and protein metabolic types do very poorly with coffee as it acts like speed in the body and over-stimulates. Kapha and carbohydrate metabolic types, who tend to have slower metabolism can typically handle a daily cup of coffee to get them going. Pitta and mixed metabolic types need to be cautious as all stimulants can imbalance and stress them.

If you are going to consume coffee, use it the way it was used back in the ninth century. Enjoy a small cup from time to time. Organic coffee in moderation does have some health benefits. The coffee bean does grow and subsist in nature after all. There is purpose for it. But fueling yourself on coffee all day or drinking one to three cups every day makes for a lifestyle that will negatively affect your health.

vegetables: raw or cooked?

Wellness practitioners continually debate whether it is best to eat vegetables cooked or raw. Some promote eating vegetables raw because they contain more nutrients while others claim the body better absorbs nutrients when vegetables are cooked (lightly steamed). In my opinion, it is best to get a good combination of both—eat half of your vegetables cooked and the other half raw.

As always, exceptions to the rule prove the rule! Broccoli, Brussels sprouts, cabbage, cauliflower, kale, mustard greens, rutabaga, turnips and watercress are among the foods that contain goitrogens, a naturally occurring chemical. Goitrogens block the production of the thyroid hormone. For those who have a sluggish metabolism, a weakened thyroid or hypothyroidism, avoid eating these foods raw! The good news is that if these foods are cooked or lightly steamed, the heat will deactivate the thiocyanate (thyroid suppressing chemical).

If you do eat these vegetables regularly (which is important because they do have extraordinary health benefits), it is essential to supplement your diet with iodine, as it is the main mineral that is needed to produce thyroid hormones. By eating iodine with these vegetables, you will counterbalance the goitrogens. The best iodine-rich food is seaweed. You can purchase seaweed (i.e. kelp, dulse, nori and hijiki) at any health food store. It can be steamed and eaten with the above vegetables, used in soups, or crushed and used as a substitute for salt. See the recipe below for a great way to incorporate seaweed into your diet.

vegetables with dulse[1]

1 cup dulse, soaked and sliced
1 carrot, cut into matchsticks
1 cup daikon, turnip or parsnip, cut into matchsticks

1 tsp sesame oil

½ tsp sea salt (optional)

1 Sauté vegetables in oil for 5–7 minutes on medium heat, or simmer until tender in ½ inch of water.
2 Add dulse and salt.
3 Cover and cook on low heat for 10 minutes.
4 Remove cover and cook off excess liquid.

Here's another exception. Foods that contain oxalic acid are better eaten cooked. Oxalic acid is a naturally occurring acid that interferes with the absorption of calcium. It is found in asparagus, beets, beet greens, chard, endive, green peppers, tomatoes and spinach. Cooking these vegetables destroys the oxalic acid which otherwise would interfere with the absorption of calcium. This does not mean that you can never eat these vegetables raw, but if you know you need to increase your calcium intake or if you have osteoporosis, choose to cook them as opposed to eating them raw.

balance and the cooked versus raw debate

Have you ever stopped to consider the seasons when choosing whether to eat vegetables raw or cooked? Think about it. In spring and summer our bodies crave salads, vegetable juices and raw vegetables, while in cooler seasons we gravitate naturally toward more cooked, steamed, roasted vegetables and soups. Heed the wisdom of the body. To maintain balance throughout the year, avoid cold and raw vegetables in the cool seasons and warming, cooked vegetables in the heat of summer.

One important note: macrobiotic diets (i.e. raw food diets) are popular with many celebrities. But before you follow the latest Hollywood trend, stop to consider where you live and where the celebrity lives. They may be living in hot climates year round where a cooling macrobiotic diet can be beneficial. If you chose to eat cold, raw vegetables in the cold winter seasons, it is unlikely that you would feel satiated. Moreover, you would contribute to dry skin and lack of insulation in your body. So it is important to consider both season and climate when choosing to eat raw or cooked foods.

Eat a good fat along with vegetables. Whether your vegetables are raw or cooked, it is important always to eat them with an essential fat. Doing so maximizes the absorption of nutrients. Beta carotene, vitamins A, K, D and E, calcium and magnesium, which are found in most vegetables, need essential fats to be absorbed and utilized by the body. So put a pat of organic butter or ghee (see Tip 19) on steamed vegetables, sprinkle ground flaxseed on soups or salads, add olives, nuts or seeds, macadamia nut oil, olive oil and/ or avocado to salads and accompany cut-up vegetables with dips such as walnut spread, hummus or guacamole.*

Finally, never microwave your vegetables. Microwaving vegetables destroys 99% of all their nutrients. Boiling destroys 66%. It is best to lightly steam vegetables because steaming destroys virtually no nutrients.

Remember, wellness does not come without balance. Exceptions aside, eating vegetables—both raw and cooked—is a perfect way to create a 50/50 balance in your nutritional lifestyle.

*All of these recipes can be found in *Putting it All Together: A Compilation of Healthy, Quick, Simple, Easy to Follow Recipes to Support You on Your Journey to Sound Nutrition* by Amy Bondar, available at the Hoffman Centre for Integrative Medicine.

"There is nothing intrinsically healthy or unhealthy about any given food. All that matters is how well a particular food or dietary regimen can fulfill your unique, genetically inherited metabolic requirements." –William Wolcott

In this day and age, we are faced with a plethora of conflicting dietary advice and an overwhelming number of food choices. We are probably more confused than ever about what to eat and why.

Nutrition is not just about "good" foods or "bad" foods, or about following the latest low-carbohydrate, high-protein diet fad. Optimum nutrition happens first at the cellular level, meaning that every morsel of food we eat has an impact on the way in which our biochemical body functions. Learning to consume the foods that promote and strengthen our body's biochemical individuality is the key to achieving optimum wellness.

How you feel today physically, mentally, emotionally and spiritually is greatly influenced by the foods you consume and the relationship between these foods and your body. A synergistic orchestration occurs at the cellular level when the body is fed the right ingredients. As a Nutritional Consulting Practitioner, it is fascinating for me to observe how slight adjustments, eliminations and additions to your nutritional lifestyles create significant transformations in how you feel, in your symptom presentation, and in your overall well being.

In my practice, it is becoming increasingly evident that one of the major causes of disease, poor health and negative symptomatic conditions is people eating against their biochemical needs. I often tell my clients that we must eat from the cells up as opposed to the mouth down. Once we start feeding the cells with the correct fuel mix, which differs for every single person, the body begins to achieve a state of balance. This is the essence of healing. Wellness does not come without balance and sound nutrition plays a fundamental role in achieving a state of balance within the body.

One of the simplest ways to determine your correct fuel mix and know with certainty that you are eating right for your body type is to keep a food journal. Write down everything you eat at each meal and then one or two hours after eating check-in with yourself. Note what is happening within your body, mind and spirit, and write that down. Include how you are feeling. You will know if you have reached your personal fuel mix if you are feeling energetic, satiated, satisfied, have good mental clarity and are free of cravings. If you do not experience this, then fine-tune your next meal by reducing or increasing your macronutrients until you have found the perfect ratios for your body.

To have certainty that your fuel mix is right for you is to understand your metabolic type and your Ayurvedic dosha (see Tips 46 and 63). These two sciences are part of my 7 Steps to Sound Nutrition™ program. Together, metabolic typing and Ayurvedic nutrition unveil how your unique body works and which specific foods are necessary to keep that body balanced and well.

There is no doubt that one person's food is another's poison. What works for one person may be detrimental to another therefore nutrition cannot be "built" for the masses. Nutrition always is about you and what your body specifically needs. Nutritional consulting—whether you are overweight, underweight, leading a healthy lifestyle, exercising regularly, experiencing disease or illness, young or aged, feeling well or fatigued—is for everyone. The more you understand your body's unique biochemical wisdom and the foods needed to fuel it to a state of balance, the more you can master optimum wellness.

Have you have been cutting eggs out of your diet because you were concerned that they would raise your cholesterol and contribute to coronary heart disease? If so, you have fallen prey to one of the biggest nutritional myths ever. Eggs have no significant effect on blood cholesterol. According to one major study, people who did not eat eggs had a higher death rate from heart attacks and strokes than those who ate eggs regularly. So my friends, get cracking!

What's the source of this nutritional myth? Much of the cholesterol research was done originally on rabbits. Since rabbits eat an entirely vegetarian diet, they could not metabolize the animal food when they were fed eggs. Their bodies did not recognize it, so their cholesterol levels increased. The estimated six-billion-dollar-cholesterol-lowering industry took those studies to the bank. Numerous studies have been done on humans, all proving that the consumption of eggs does not affect blood cholesterol or the risk of developing coronary heart disease. There is actually one documented case of a man who ate twenty to thirty eggs a day for fifteen years, and his cholesterol levels were always in normal range!

Eggs are one of nature's most perfect foods. In *The Nutritional Bypass: Reverse Atherosclerosis Without Surgery,* Dr. David Rowland states, "eggs are the healthiest food on the planet. They provide protein of the highest quality plus all known vitamins and minerals (except vitamin C)".[1] Eggs are especially rich in vitamins A, D and B1, niacin, phosphorus, calcium, the most absorbable form of iron, sulphur and the amino acids tryptophan and methionine (a powerful antioxidant). They are also an excellent source of omega-3 fatty acids, especially DHA. DHA is necessary for mental development, so eggs are excellent for pregnant women as well as for infants four months and older. In Asia, eggs are considered a brain food.

Eggs do have cholesterol (220mg per egg), but it is the good cholesterol that the body recognizes and needs. Cholesterol is essential for many bodily processes. As Rowland notes, it is in every cell of every body. It is used to conduct nerve impulses, make bile, produce hormones, synthesize vitamin D and ensure optimal functioning of the nervous system. As Sally Fallon writes in *Nourishing Traditions,* "egg yolks are the most concentrated source of choline, which is necessary for keeping the cholesterol moving in the blood stream."[2]

The body produces 70% of its own cholesterol and gets the other 30% from foods. When the body gets enough of the beneficial cholesterol from whole, natural foods such as eggs, it stops producing its own. In *The Cholesterol Myths,* Dr. Uffe Ravnskov explains that in many studies, "those who ate the smallest amount of cholesterol had the highest levels of blood cholesterol."[3] When you eat less cholesterol, your liver makes more on its own. As Gary Null states in *The Complete Encyclopedia of Natural Healing,* "your liver is a cholesterol-making machine, able to churn up 1500 mg a day, six times what you would normally eat."[4] So lowering the good cholesterol foods such as eggs may actually increase your body's production of the bad cholesterol!

It is oxidized cholesterol that is bad for us, not the beneficial cholesterol found in eggs and other whole foods. The body does not recognize oxidized cholesterol; as a result the bad cholesterol in the blood rises. Oxidized cholesterol is found in deep fried foods such as French Fries, hydrogenated oils found in most manufactured and processed foods, and in foods that have been altered from their natural state such as powdered eggs and milk.

Sally Fallon makes an interesting note about Egg Beaters® as she cites a study that looked at rats that were fed fresh eggs compared to rats that were fed Egg Beaters®. The study found that rats that were fed fresh eggs thrived, were perfectly healthy, and grew normally. The rats that were fed Egg Beaters® did not grow normally; they were stunted, and all died long before reaching maturity.

It is important to know that all eggs are not equal. When shopping, choose free range, organic eggs. Also look for eggs from hens or chickens that were fed flax or fishmeal or that were pasture fed. This will increase the omega-3 ratios in the eggs (see Tip 53). This is extremely important because as Fallon states, "in chickens only fed grains, the omega-3:6 ratio is extremely imbalanced. Omega-6 can be as much as nineteen times higher than omega-3s"[5]. This imbalance is harmful to our health—the balanced ratio of omega-3:6 should be 1:4.

Incorporate whole eggs into your daily nutritional lifestyle and have no fear because they will not affect your cholesterol levels. It is sugar, high-carbohydrate diets, junk foods and eating against your metabolic type that are the real culprits for high cholesterol in the blood. As long as you are not sensitive or allergic to them, eggs will only support you as you journey toward optimum wellness.

Here's a final interesting note on cholesterol... Cholesterol levels in the blood naturally fluctuate throughout the day. They also vary from season to season, and are especially higher in the winter months. So if you are getting your cholesterol checked, perhaps it is wise and useful to have it checked at different times in different months before forming any definitive conclusions. Nutrition can play a significant role in raising and lowering cholesterol levels, so before jumping into taking drugs that can have harmful side effects, especially on the liver, seek out a qualified Nutritional Consulting Practitioner (i.e., me!) that can help you make necessary nutritional adjustments.

The origin of the word "nightshade" is not clear, but some historians say that it was referred to in old English writings as "evil and loving nature of the night." Others say the name originated among the Romans, who ground up a deadly black nightshade and put it in an alcoholic drink intended for the enemy. There are even reports that animals grazing in fields where nightshades grew were often found crippled or dead.

The Solonaceae family—the "deadly nightshades"—include: banana pepper, bell pepper, belladonna, capsicum, cayenne, chili pepper, curry, eggplant, paprika, peppers, pimento, potato, Tabasco, tobacco and tomato. Black pepper, sweet potato and yam are not included as they are a part of other botanical families.

Dr. Sherry A. Rogers explains in *Pain Free in 6 Weeks,* that the nightshades contain potent alkaloids. In fact, some of the alkaloids are so potent that they are used to make medicinal prescriptive drugs and harmful, toxic pesticides. The alkaloid solanine, abundant in the nightshades, is a calcium and sodium inhibitor. This is significant for those with arthritis, osteoporosis, chronic pain and other inflammatory conditions because calcium's fundamental roles are to maintain strong healthy bones and to regulate the contraction and relaxation of the muscles. Another alkaloid, glycoalkaloid, interferes with the function of the enzyme that makes nerves and muscles work properly.

Nightshades are the most abundantly consumed vegetable family in North America. Potatoes are the number one vegetable eaten, followed by the tomato. I find it fascinating that over 80 million people in North America suffer from arthritis and other inflammatory conditions. I have no doubt that there is a positive correlation between the two.

Alkaloids ingested from the nightshades silently accumulate in your system until they reach a high enough dose to produce pain. You may have eaten nightshades throughout your life, but not acquire the symptomatology until years later. It is also important to note that sensitivities and genetic predisposition to inflammatory conditions vary from person to person. Some people may experience pain after eating tomatoes but be okay with peppers, whereas others might become inflamed after eating potatoes but no other nightshade creates any symptoms.

Rogers has found that "over 74–90% of the people who ache and hurt, regardless of their diagnostic label or type, have sensitivity to nightshades."[1] When all the nightshades are completely eliminated from the diet, many such symptoms disappear. When the nightshades are re-introduced, the inflammation and pain begins again.

If you have any type of inflammatory condition, I highly recommend the elimination of all nightshades for a period of three months. After that time, try incorporating some back into the diet and see if it makes a difference in how you feel. And remember, even a little bit during your elimination trial can be too much. If you do in fact notice a difference and pain starts again, it is wise to keep all nightshades completely out of your diet indefinitely.

Finally, read the list of ingredients on everything you buy, as these foods, especially the spices, tomatoes and potatoes (including their powders and starches) are hidden in sauces, packaged foods, etc. Also watch supplements, as some contain cayenne, potato or tomato.

The most important nutrient in your body is plain water. Basic bio-chemistry tells us that bones are one-quarter water, the muscles are three-quarters water, the brain is 76% water and the blood that carries your nutrients is 82% water.

Dr. Joseph Mercola explains,

> Water is essential for digestion, nutrient absorption and assimilation. It aids in circulation, helps regulate the body's temperature, lubricates and cushions the joints, keeps skin healthy and helps remove toxins from the body.[1]

The quality of your tissues and the functioning of your cells is not only dependent on the amount of water you drink but also on the quality of water you drink.

There is a great deal of conflicting information on which water source is better for your health: tap, filtered, distilled, reverse osmosis, well water or pure spring water. After sifting through and making sense of some of this research, I have come to conclude that clean reverse osmosis filtered water and pure spring water are the safest and best choices.

With certainty we can say that tap water is absolutely the worst source. Chlorine and fluoride are extremely toxic to the body. In fact, fluoride is so toxic it is used as a rat poison and pesticide. Also consider the pipes through which the water travels. Most pipes contain lead, which is another extreme heavy metal toxin that may contribute to cardiovascular disease and cancer. The Colgan Institute found there are "over 60,000 chemical contaminants in water. Any municipal water supply harbors at least 1000."[2] The report also revealed that of the 954 city water supplies tested,

30% were seriously contaminated. Drinking tap water will not kill you, but ingesting toxic fluids day after day will indeed pollute your cells, muscles, organs and brain and will prevent you from achieving a state of optimum wellness.

Distilled water is not your best source either. It is highly acidic. Most of us already have high acidity in our bodies, so compounding this with acidic water, is pushing your pH in the wrong direction. At one time, many people promoted distilled water because it was said to be free of contaminants, but as Mercola reports, "many of the devices that distill the water are made of metals and actually add certain toxic metals, like nickel, into the water."[3] Moreover, distilled water can actually leach minerals out of your bloodstream.

A reverse osmosis filter is highly recommended, so you can be sure that the above contaminants will be filtered out of your water. Reverse osmosis does de-mineralize water, but the amount of minerals absorbed from water is so minimal that this is not a real concern. You will get more minerals by having a sound nutritional lifestyle loaded with mineral rich fruits, vegetables, gluten-free whole grains and protein, and taking supplements, than you will by drinking mineralized water.

As for clean, pure spring water, just ensure you know that your source is a real spring! As Mercola states, "40% of the bottled waters on the market are not from a spring but a tap (including popular brands such as Dasani, Evian and Aquafina)."[4] At the Hoffman Centre for Integrative Medicine we recommend and trust drinking Monashee Spring Water (www.monasheespringwater.com). This water is straight from the heart of the Canadian Rocky Mountains. It is alkaline water with a pH of 7–7 ½. It also is ozonized and has virtually no fluoride.

According to Dr. Mercola, the only down side to drinking bottled spring water is that the plastic bottles can leach an unsafe chemical called BPA. He states "BPA can cause genetic abnormalities and exhibits hormone-like properties, imitating the effects of naturally occurring estrogens."[5] On the bottom of the plastic bottles there is a triangle with a number in it. The #7 is a better plastic, as there is less chemical leaching. Anything less than #7 should be avoided (Monashee uses # 7 plastics). It is best to drink from glass bottles and switch to high-density polyethylene Nalgene bottles that you can buy at most trekking and outside adventure stores such as North Face and Mountain Equipment Co-op.

Don't forget to always clean your water bottles. They can carry numerous strains of bacteria and germs. And for the sake of those around you, when filling your water bottles don't put the rim of your bottle too close to the water spout. Doing so can pass on many germs and bacteria.

We have always been told that we should drink eight to ten glasses of water a day. The standard is that for every fifty pounds of body weight, you should drink one litre of water. But as with everything in nutrition, one size does not fit all. Some body types (e.g. kapha types, see Tip 46) need less water as they retain water easily and already have a lot of moisture in their bodies. Those who work out regularly need to drink more water than the sedentary person. One of the best ways to gauge how much water you need is by looking at the color of your urine. A deep yellow color usually means that you are not drinking enough (note that B vitamins will also make your urine this yellow, so it may be difficult to tell). Ideally, your urine should be clear or a pale yellow.

Finally, avoid drinking cold water. Cold water reduces the pulse rate, increases arterial tension, raises body temperature, increases urine flow and stays in the stomach longer than warm water, affecting optimal digestion. Avoid drinking large amounts of water at one time, particularly at meals, because this can over-strain the muscles of the digestive tract. Actually, it's best to drink water before or after a meal, as opposed to during the meal. Most importantly, do not wait until you are thirsty to drink. If you are thirsty, it means that you are dehydrated. Sipping water throughout the day is the best way to stay hydrated and to ensure you are getting just the right amount of water for your body type.

here comes the sun...

"What nature delivers to us is never stale. Because what nature creates has eternity in it." –Isaac Bashevis Singer

As summer is just around the corner, it is time once again to adjust our diets. According to John Douillard, in *The 3-Season Diet,* "summer is a time of high energy, demanding the energy-producing properties of fruits, vegetables and other [fibrous and complex] carbs."[1]

If we were cyclically mindful, strictly following a seasonal diet and in tune with what we eat from season to season, the summer would naturally be the time to eat a high-carbohydrate diet (whereas in the winter our bodies are more conducive to a low-carbohydrate diet). This is not to say that you should go crazy on carbohydrates in the summer. As I say all the time, we all need different amounts and types of foods for our biochemical individuality, as well as specific health conditions. But with the longer hours, hotter weather and higher levels of activity, the body naturally gravitates to more cooling, sweeter and refreshing fruits and vegetables at this time of year.

The grocery stores are full of luscious, juicy and colorful fruits in the summer, but note this produce is mostly imported. It is best to get most of your produce locally grown at health food stores and at farmer's markets. While this might not leave us with many tropical options, it does provide us with foods that connect us to our environment and climate.

The following is a list of produce that is best to buy and eat for each summer month. Just because some of your favorites may not be on these lists, it does not mean you cannot have them just know that these lists comprise what is most available and grown in accordance to our seasonal temperature.

June: asparagus, broccoli, cherries, green onions, lettuce, peas, radishes, rhubarb and strawberries.

July: beans, beets, broccoli, cabbage, carrots, cauliflower, corn, cucumbers, green onions, lettuce, peas, peppers, radishes, raspberries, rhubarb, Saskatoon berries, strawberries and summer squash.

August: beans, beets, broccoli, cabbage, carrots, cauliflower, celery, corn, cucumbers, lettuce, onions, peas, peppers, pumpkin, radishes, raspberries, rhubarb, rutabagas, Saskatoon berries, strawberries, summer squash, tomatoes and winter squash.

If you are eating grains, summer is the best time to bring oats back into the diet. Also, the best oils for this season are butter, ghee (clarified butter), coconut, olive and sunflower. Focus on lighter, lower fat proteins such as chicken breast, turkey breast, Cornish hen, legumes and white fish. As for spices, the cooling sweeter tastes are ideal such as coriander, mint, cardamom and fennel. In general, summer is the time to promote sweet (through fruits, essential fats and proteins—not sugar!), bitter (arugula, fiddleheads, spring mix, Brussel sprouts) and astringent (cranberries, beans and tea) tastes over spicy, salty and sour tastes.

The start of every season is always exciting. I urge you to use it as an opportunity to purchase new foods, create more variety in your lifestyle, try new summer recipes, shop at different markets and savor some of the tastes you have been waiting for all year. The start of every season is also an ideal time to come in for a follow-up session to fine-tune your nutrition based on your individual needs.

Many of you often ask me if I put you on a low-carbohydrate diet. It may seem like it because I often recommend the elimination of all sugar, grains (especially gluten-grains), grain flours and refined foods. However, you can be certain that you are in fact still eating carbohydrates. The difference is you are only eating the safest and healthiest ones.

By now, we know the difference between refined and complex carbohydrates. But there are more important classifications of carbohydrates, and to achieve optimum wellness through sound nutrition, it is important to understand the significant difference between them. Dr. Loren Cordain differentiates between two groups of carbohydrates in his eye-opening book, *The Paleolithic Diet*. Paleocarbs include vegetables, fruits and some tubers such as squash, pumpkin and sweet potato. Neocarbs (carbohydrates introduced in the last 10,000 years or less), include grains, legumes and flour products, which have not existed for most of human history.

Cordain explains, "Since 99.99% of our genes were formed before the development of agriculture, from a biological perspective, we are still hunter-gatherers."[1] From a biochemical point of view, this means that our bodies are physiologically unable to recognize and fully digest and metabolize grains and flours and, as a result the rate of metabolic disease in this country has skyrocketed.

For the past thirty years, we have been misguided, ill informed and at the mercy of the pyramid food guides, where we have been told that grain-based, high neo-carbohydrate diets are good for us. These food guides are predominately built around neocarbs. Six to eleven servings of grains, breads, pastas, cereals, etc. a day has, without a doubt, significantly contributed to the highest rate of obesity, Type II diabetes, insulin resistance, high cholesterol and high triglycerides this nation has ever seen. It is interesting to note that it was the Department of Agriculture that developed the Canada Food Guide (the base of the pyramid does suggest a financial political interest stronger than an interest in the health of Canadians).

Dr. Allan Spreen sums it up perfectly, as he states,

> The huge base of the so-called Food Pyramid; that moronic image from government bureaucrats, is in large part responsible for the unimaginable amount of obesity rampant in this country.[2]

Grains and flours contain antinutrients, which are naturally occurring chemical compounds that protect crops from predators. Processing and cooking does not rid the grains of these chemicals, making them abundant in our diets and bodies. As a result, these antinutrients can create allergies and undermine the integrity of the digestive lining. No wonder so many people are allergic to gluten (the protein of wheat, rye, barley, spelt and kamut). Health begins in the colon, so if grains have compromised the integrity of the digestive system, a host of other problems throughout the body will likely result.

Another affect of grains is molecular mimicry. When foreign proteins (grains, viruses, bacteria, etc.) enter the body, a "mistaken identity" occurs because proteins in the tissues of the body resemble the foreign proteins. The immune system cannot differentiate between its self-proteins and the foreign proteins. As a result, "when the immune system defends the body against such foreign proteins, as it is supposed to, it also attacks the very similar self-proteins."[3] For those with a genetic predisposition, this creates an inflammatory response in the body and many autoimmune diseases such as multiple sclerosis, cancer, celiac disease, Type I diabetes and rheumatoid arthritis.

So it is not that I am eliminating grains, grain flours and sugars (the neocarbs) to follow the "high-protein/low-carb" craze. Rather, I am doing it to protect your health, to prevent and aid in the reversal of autoimmune diseases and metabolic syndromes, and to move your bodies to an optimum state of wellness with the paleocarbs, which the body was genetically designed to fuel on.

If you have upper respiratory conditions, anemia, fatigue, bowel complaints, Syndrome X (obesity, Type II diabetes, high cholesterol, high triglycerides, insulin resistance), autoimmune conditions, diseases of the nervous system or the mind, try eliminating the neocarbs and see if any of the symptoms improve.

I am not saying that all grains are "bad," but we can all benefit from vastly reducing grains. It is important to note that if your body is in a state of balance, if your diet and lifestyle are optimized and if you do not have a predisposition to autoimmune disease, minimal gluten-free grains (brown rice, wild rice, buckwheat, millet, quinoa, amaranth and oats) would likely be okay for your body. In general, without determining your unique body type, half a cup (for women) and one cup (for men) serving of cooked whole grains a day, as opposed to six to eleven servings a day is a huge difference. But in my practice, the results speak for themselves: significant reversal of symptoms, dramatic weight loss and improvements in health and overall well being are seen as soon as we eliminate the neocarbs from diets. Bottom line, your carbohydrate consumption should predominately be coming from fibrous vegetables and fruit.

As I remind you all the time, we must take into account biochemical individuality. Some body types can handle more grains than others, and some need more carbohydrates than others. The types of paleocarbs differ from person to person as well. All fruits and vegetables are not assimilated equally in each of our bodies, so it is essential to understand which ones are right for you. Take pride in the fact that you are eating the safer carbohydrates, that you are not apart of the "low-carb" craze and that your nutritional lifestyles will help journey your body to a state of optimum wellness.

If you would like some more information on this nutrition tip, I highly recommend reading:

- *The No Grain Diet,* by Dr. Joseph Mercola
- *The Paleolithic Diet,* by Dr. Loren Cordain
- *Dangerous Grains,* by James Braly and Ron Hoggan

After finishing a very garlicky Caesar salad, I felt the need to do some experimenting on how to naturally get the lingering and potent taste of garlic out of my mouth. In so doing this, I came up with this nutrition tip!

I do not recommend restaurant after-dinner mints. Typically, they are full of sugar, artificial flavors and food dye. I also do not trust any foods that do not have a list of ingredients on the wrappers, because you never quite know what you are ingesting.

I also advise my clients to avoid chewing gum for three reasons. First, it is full of aspartame and other harmful artificial sweeteners, food coloring, synthetic chemicals such as BHT and BHA and artificial flavors. Second, for those with mercury amalgams, chewing gum has been well documented by Dr. Joseph Mercola, to release more mercury from fillings into the bloodstream. Third, when you chew gum, your pancreas is stimulated and releases the digestive enzymes that aid in the digestive process. When you chew a lot of gum throughout the day, these essential enzymes are depleted and wasted and the ability to effectively break down and absorb food when you do have a meal, is compromised.

And then there is mouthwash—seeing as how it is considered a household poison, we won't even go there!

So, my experiment was quite simple. I went into my spice/herb cupboard to see what I could find. I happened to have just bought cinnamon sticks to boil for a sweet aroma in my house, so I thought I'd break off a piece to see if that would help. For an intense aftertaste of garlic, it didn't quite do the job, but I would say that it would be beneficial for a general sweetening of the breath. It is also important to note, that cinnamon is excellent for diabetes, insulin resistance or hypoglycemia as it helps control insulin levels. Chewing on some cinnamon after a meal or sprinkling ground cinnamon on foods would be an excellent therapeutic thing to do for those with compromised blood sugars.

I then tried fennel seeds, as I remembered they are served in many East Indian restaurants after the meal. I began to chew on about thirty seeds for approximately 5 minutes and the strong anise (licorice) taste overpowered the garlic. After doing some reading on fennel, I realized that the seeds are also served at East Indian restaurants to help aid in the digestive process. As explained in *Nutritional Herbology* by Mark Pederson, fennel stimulates the pancreas to increase the secretion of digestive enzymes resulting in more efficient and effective digestion and less flatulence. Medicinally they have been used for centuries to help relieve gastrointestinal complaints, flatulence and cramping.

I highly recommend that before grabbing unnatural and harmful gum, mints or mouth wash, you buy some fennel seeds, cinnamon or fresh mint leaves and keep them in your home, office, wallet or purse for whenever you may need your breath to feel fresh, clean and healthy.

The following are some other natural breath fresheners:

- Peppy-Mint Breath Refresher by Aveda
- Peppermint Breath Drops by Burt's Bees
- Natural Mouthwash with Aloe by Tom's of Maine

Nutrition is just like anything else in life. It is a journey with ups and downs, twists and turns, the expected and unexpected, the challenge and the ease. It is not about perfection or failure; it is about embracing all that is to come on your journey.

We put a great deal of pressure on ourselves when it comes to our food choices. Many people feel guilt or beat themselves up if they fall off their plan, if they eat "bad" foods or foods they know they should avoid. Striving to have a perfect diet or being excessively meticulous about following your nutritional lifestyles often exaggerates these feelings.

What you do 90–95% of the time is what counts. If you have thirty days in a month, you typically have four to play with. Rather than feeling bad about those few times that you journey down a different road, use them as lessons. Tap into how you feel after you eat something that you know you should be avoiding. Many people often realize the significant power food has over the health of the human body when they do. For example, one of my clients told me that she had not touched sugar in weeks and one day she had some dessert and felt absolutely horrible. She experienced all the symptoms she had before she came in to work with me. It was a great realization for her to know how awful sugar and dairy really made her feel. Other people realize how tired or lethargic they get after having a meal with pasta or bread when they had been avoiding it for some time.

We often don't realize or connect with how food makes us feel or that many of our symptoms may be due to eating foods that go against our metabolic body types. But when you begin to make these connections it is quite inspiring and motivating to continue on your nutritional journey. So, instead of giving up after you've hit a road block, or after the unexpected happens or when your

tempation overrides your willpower, acknowledge how it made you
feel, look at the drawbacks and blessings you received from the
experience, transcend it and keep going.

If you have been off your nutritional path for a while, there is no
reason why you can't continue on. It's not about starting over; it's
about a new day. Like everything else in life you just have to keep
on keepin' on.

Sushi has become an eating hot spot over the years and though there are some health benefits to eating it, there are some drawbacks as well. The following are some important tips to consider when eating out and to ensure your sushi experience is as nutritionally sound and healthy as possible.

Go for the sashimi (raw fish). This will ensure you avoid the refined white rice, which converts to glucose quickly in the body, affecting blood sugars and insulin levels, and inevitably causing weight gain. White rice is stripped of all its minerals making it an acidic food and because it is sticky rice it will also be mucous forming, likely contributing to a stuffed nose or a throat needing to be cleared. The rice is also sweetened with cane sugar, so for those watching your sugar intake, be cautious. If you can't deal with the raw fish on its own (which is understandable!), then at least take half of the rice off each piece. You will be surprised at how much rice is left over on your plate! Finally, more and more sushi restaurants are now serving brown rice so if it were available, the brown rice would be a better choice.

Hand rolls are an excellent choice. They contain less rice and have the most nori (seaweed). Nori is rich in iodine, which is the main mineral needed to help produce the thyroid hormone. Nori will help speed up metabolism and increase energy. It is also high in vitamin B12 making it an excellent food for vegetarians. You can ask for extra sheets of nori and eat it with your sashimi in place of the rice.

Be cautious of soy sauce. It is really important to read the ingredients on all soy sauce as most contain wheat, monosodium glutamate (MSG) and high levels of sodium, which many of us are sensitive to. The best thing to do is bring your own tamari (wheat-free soy sauce which can be bought at any health food store) from home.

Though I don't recommend eating soy, fermented soy is okay in moderation and provides beneficial bacteria for the gut, which can fight the rare possibility of getting parasites from eating raw fish. So the soy sauce (if it is pure) and the miso soup are excellent to incorporate into your sushi meal. It is actually recommended to drink miso soup before you eat any sushi to prepare the digestive system for the meal.

Stay away from the deep fried foods such as tempura. Deep-fried is deep-fried. Enough said!

Drink plenty of green tea. It is full of antioxidants and many sushi restaurants use "real" green tea, which is more potent than a commercial tea bag.

Try to not overdo the pickled ginger, as that too is full of sugar. The wasabi however is pure (ideally!).

One of the most important things you can do when eating sushi is to avoid the highest mercury containing fish—shark, swordfish, red snapper and tuna steak. The safest ones to stick to are shrimp, wild Alaskan salmon, trout, flounder and fish roe.

Ensure you are choosing high quality sushi restaurants where you can be sure the fish is fresh and prepared properly.

A great benefit to eating sushi is that you receive an abundance of essential fats from the fish and avocado. Some rolls now come with black olives, which increase the "good" fat content even more. These fats are essential for our health and are a must at each meal we eat. They are often not incorporated regularly in many restaurants so this is definitely a bonus for frequenting sushi joints.

It is easy to over-order at a sushi restaurant. Though the pieces look small, they are extremely filling, especially with all the rice. Start with a small bowl of miso soup, reduce the rice rolls, order more hand cones and choose more sashimi over sushi.

Finally, consider making your own sushi as a snack for home or to pack in your kids' lunches: nori, brown rice, avocado and smoked wild salmon (lox) make a perfect roll. It doesn't need to be fancy or perfectly rolled, it just needs to be healthy and taste good!

So enjoy going for sushi from time to time, just be a little more conscious and aware of how and what you are ordering to ensure your sushi experience is a healthy one.

In the past year I have been increasingly recommending the use of coconut oil as part of your daily nutritional lifestyles. As I always say, eating what grows and subsists in nature is one of the fundamental keys to achieving optimum wellness and coconut is no exception. A wonder food from the palm tree, a fruit from the gods, coconut and its oil have incredible health benefits. As Dr. Joseph Mercola has listed in many of his articles (which can be found at www.mercola.com), coconut oil can:

- Help you lose weight, or maintain your already healthy weight,
- Reduce your risk of heart disease,
- Lower your cholesterol,
- Improve conditions for those with diabetes and chronic fatigue,
- Improve Crohn's disease, IBS and other digestive disorders,
- Prevent other disease and general illness with its powerful antibacterial, antiviral and antifungal agents,
- Increase metabolism and promote healthy thyroid function,
- Boost your daily energy and
- Rejuvenate your skin and prevent wrinkles.

It is true that coconut oil has saturated fat, but saturated fat is not as detrimental to our health as we have been led to believe. In fact, coconut oil is comprised of the safest and healthiest of the saturated fats. Two-thirds of the oil is made up of medium-chain fatty acids which are easily digested, increase metabolism, maximize energy and promote weight loss. These medium-chain fatty acids are also the most stable of the saturated fats. When heated and stored at room temperature, coconut oil does not turn into harmful trans-fatty acids, oxidize or create oxidative stress in the body like most polyunsaturated vegetable oils do, especially soybean oil.

The medium-chain fatty acids are also used differently in the body than other oils. Rather than being stored in the body's cells, they go directly to the liver where the oil is converted into energy. "When you eat coconuts and coconut oil your body uses it immediately to make energy rather than store it as body fat."[1] This energy production speeds up metabolism, triggering weight loss and increases body temperature, hormone production, thyroid activity and overall energy expenditure in the body. This is especially important and beneficial for those with low thyroid function or hypothyroidism.

For diabetics, this increase in metabolism is crucial because it helps regulate blood sugar levels. Dr. Mercola explains, "as metabolism increases, it stimulates the production of needed insulin and increases absorption of glucose into cells, thus helping both Type I and Type II diabetics."[2]

Coconut oil also contains lauric and monolaurin fatty acids that have antiviral, antifungal and antibacterial properties. These fatty acids help boost the body's immunity and can help kill herpes, Epstein-Barr viruses, candida and giardia. This is especially important for people with chronic fatigue syndrome (CFS) as the key to overcoming CFS is strengthening the body's immune system and ridding it of any harmful pathogens, viruses or bacteria.

Dr. Ray Peat, a physiologist, also explains that the antimicrobial properties of the fatty acids promote intestinal health by killing microorganisms that may cause chronic inflammation in the digestive tract. Coconut oil can soothe inflammation and help heal the lining of the digestive system for those with irritable bowel syndrome or Crohn's disease.

Coconut oil is also wonderful for skin health. It is absorbed into the skin and the cellular structure of the connective tissues, making for a more youthful and glowing look. More importantly, it prevents liver spots, blemishes, sun spots and wrinkles.

Coconut oil can be used for all cooking, as a spread on toast, melted on steamed vegetables or added to your protein shakes. It is high in protein, low in carbohydrates and is an excellent source of folic acid, all B vitamins, calcium, magnesium and potassium.

It is important to consider the source when you buy coconut oil. Ensure there is no trans-fatty oils added, it has not been genetically modified and it is organic. At the Hoffman Centre for Integrative Medicine, we trust, sell and promote Extra Virgin Coconut Oil by Garden of Life, or you can look for Tropical Traditions Virgin Coconut Oil at any health food store. Coconut oil is more expensive than most oils (ranging from $15–$24) so if you are finding less expensive brands it is likely not high quality oil. Always store your coconut oil at room temperature and its shelf life is five years so you definitely receive value when buying a more expensive, better quality brand.

snack attack!

There is a common experience among us all—the mid-morning and mid-afternoon crash. Fatigue sets in, energy drops, concentration is sub-optimal, coffee and sugar cravings are overriding your willpower, you feel you could snap at the next person who walks through the door, your stomach is feeling hollow and you swear the vending machine and Starbucks are calling your name. I like to call it the "snack attack!"

Wellness does not come without balance. One of the easiest ways to achieve a state of balance in the body throughout the day is to eat regularly and incorporate small mid-morning and mid-afternoon snacks. For many people, snacking is essential to balance blood sugars, trigger metabolism for weight loss, to prevent sugar cravings and to avoid over-eating at meal times.

Some body types do not feel the need for snacks. These types typically have slower metabolisms and can go for a longer period of time without eating. Those with fast metabolisms however, or those with Type II diabetes, hypoglycemia or who want to burn body fat, must ensure they eat more frequently. Listen to your body. If you are feeling hungry, your energy is dropping, you are feeling scattered, you are getting irritable, impatient or moody, your mental acuity is lacking, or your blood sugars are dropping, then it is essential to plan for and enjoy a small snack.

It is important however to be mindful of what you are choosing for snacks. Most people gravitate towards refined carbohydrates/sugar, which is counterproductive to trying to maintain balance in the body. Protein bars with many hidden sugars and soy, coffee, muffins, crackers, sweetened yogurts, bread, chips, cookies and other baked goods are the worst foods you can put into your body when the "snack attack" sets in.

There are always healthy options and foods that you can bring
with you to work, school, or to keep at your office, in your car or
purse, and carry with you if you are on-the-go. Be organized, plan
ahead and always have the right foods available in your kitchen.
Snacks should be planned into your nutritional lifestyles with as
much attention as your main meals are. When planning snacks
it is wise to focus on fibrous carbohydrates, protein and essential
fats. This balance of macronutrients will keep your blood sugars
stable, keep you satiated, prevent sugar cravings and maximize
your energy.

The following is a list of healthy, quick and portable snacks:

- Celery with almond butter
- Fresh vegetable juice with a teaspoon of hazelnut butter
- Plain yogurt with ground flaxseed, walnuts and berries
- 3 tablespoons of raw, unsalted nuts or seeds and a piece
  of fruit
- Half an avocado
- Cut up vegetables with hummus, guacamole or
  walnut spread*
- Nori roll-ups (slices of oven roasted chicken or turkey rolled
  with avocado, spinach and cucumber)
- Cottage cheese and cinnamon
- Celery, cucumber or peppers with a slice of mozza-
  rella cheese
- Bowl of soup with ground flaxseed or hemp seed
- Olives
- Protein shake
- Apple with almond or cashew butter
- Hard boiled egg
- Nutmegs*

- Nutaroons*
- Piña colada chewies*
- Quick halvah*
- Zucchini muffins*
- 100% manna or sprouted bread with a tablespoon of nut butter or hummus
- Half a cup of chickpeas or other beans with crushed dulse or kelp (seaweeds)
- Turkey, beef or buffalo jerky (MSG-free)
- Raincoast crackers (healthy crackers found at Sunterra Market, the Red Tree and Second to None Meats) with sliced avocado or nut butter
- Shot of wheatgrass and a tablespoon of almonds or walnuts
- Fresh coconut chunks
- Half a can wild salmon or sardines
- Half a chicken breast
- Piece of fruit or dried fruit
- Trail mix (flax, walnuts, almonds, coconut and carob)
- Baked seaweed chips

*These snacks can be found in *Putting it All Together: A Compilation of Healthy, Quick, Simple, Easy to Follow Recipes to Support You on Your Journey to Sound Nutrition* by Amy Bondar, available at the Hoffman Centre for Integrative Medicine.

"Your body is the vehicle you have been given to carry you through life, and it feels better to be in a healthy body than in an unhealthy one!" –Christina Brown

Often people have a great challenge with weight loss or following through with their nutritional programs. They will stick with a program for a short period of time and then find themselves falling right back into old patterns and feelings of defeat and frustration. They know what they need to do to lose weight or change their diets, but can't seem to find the motivation or inspiration to put the principles into practice. This struggle is not due to a lack of willpower, diligence, motivation or dedication, because as Dr. John Demartini says, "you will be wilful and inspired to do what is intended if it aligns with your highest values."[1]

It is important to define your values and understand what is most important to you.

1   Make a list of the following values: spiritual, religious, mental, vocational, financial, familial and other relationships, social and physical.
2   Determine which of these values are most important to you; rank them from highest to lowest. If you are not sure what your highest values are consider, what it is that you spend most of your time, money or energy on, what you think or talk about the most and what you feel most deeply about.
3   Once you have your value list, begin linking weight loss or creating a sound nutritional lifestyle to your highest values (this exercise can be done for each value, not only your highest). Ask yourself the following questions:

- How will losing weight and/or creating a sound nutritional lifestyle affect my relationships with my family?
- How will losing weight and/or creating a sound nutritional lifestyle better my business?
- How will losing weight and/or creating a sound nutritional lifestyle help me meet my financial goals?
- How will losing weight and/or creating a sound nutritional lifestyle improve my mental state and thirst for knowledge and wisdom?
- How will losing weight and/or creating a sound nutritional lifestyle transform my social life?
- How will losing weight and/or creating a sound nutritional lifestyle support my physical health?
- How will losing weight and/or creating a sound nutritional lifestyle affect my spiritual or religious practice?

4 Create a list of reasons for each value and fill an entire page or more, until you reach a moment of deep realization, inspiration and a tear in your eye. Write enough reasons until you feel in your heart that losing weight and creating a sound nutritional lifestyle will enhance the things you value the most in your life. And by not reaching your weight loss goals or implementing the sound nutritional lifestyle you will hinder the things that mean the most to you.

There is no shortcut to this exercise. In your mind you might read this and see that it is logical and say that you get it, but it is in your heart where you must feel it and experience that moment of inspiration to make the changes you desire. It is only by writing out every single detail and envisioning each detail that transformation and inspiration will come. At the back of this book there is a designated page devoted to helping you complete this exercise. I urge you to take the time to do this so you have the purpose to create and maintain your sound nutritional lifestyle. If you still struggle with this exercise on your own, make an appointment with me so we can work through it together.

It is also important to note, that you may not meet your weight loss goals or change your nutritional lifestyles because you are receiving more benefits out of your current lifestyle and eating patterns than you are drawbacks. But once you realize that you are getting more drawbacks than benefits from eating the way you are, that is the moment you become inspired and wilful to make the changes you desire.

I urge you to dig deep. Spend time understanding and realizing what is most important to you in your life. I hope you all have a moment of inspiration and truly see how weight loss or creating a sound nutritional lifestyle can be a vehicle in actualizing the things that you value the most.

The following is an example of one of my clients who linked losing weight to her highest values:

how weight loss supports my "highest values" and goals

- It will require a new level of dedication and faith to do this—Faith
- I believe that overeating is a sin—putting away with that sin will have spiritual rewards—Faith
- Leaning on my God for strength and solutions to my problems instead of on food to make me feel better will help me grow spiritually—Faith
- I will be able to feed my family much better—and hopefully have my son avoid my fate with weight—Family
- I will have more energy to keep up with my son and do stuff with him—Family

- I bet I'll have a better sex life/husband more interested —Marriage
- I will be able to sit in the Mustang better—it's NOT made for fat people—Marriage
- My knees and ankles will stop hurting when I walk—My Dogs/Health
- It will be easier for the dogs to pull me in the sulky—My Dogs
- Maybe my allergies will clear up (with less milk products and toxins)—Health
- My acne may also clear up (with less milk products and toxins)—Health
- I will have reduced intestinal problems once I can balance my fibre and listen to my body's needs throughout "the month"—Health
- I can do sports I enjoy—i.e. skiing—Health/Fun
- I will be able to do "normal" things more comfortably—air plane seats, stampede rides, horseback riding, etc.—Fun
- I will be able to take up jogging again (I love jogging!) —Fun/Health
- I will have much, much more energy!—Health
- Losing weight will support my health—Health
- I will be healthier and live longer—Health
- I will be able to enjoy life much more without having to constantly worry about what I'm eating, when I can eat next and what to make every day—Faith/Health
- I will be able to shop in normal stores, and can enjoy buying matching clothes that I like, not just clothes that fit. I Love shopping!—Fun
- People won't judge me for making my dogs haul my fat butt around instead of walking—Self Esteem

- My family and friends will be proud of me (and this is a reason I'd love to do it without surgery)—Self Esteem/ Family/Relationships
- I will achieve one of my life-long goals—Self Esteem/ Spirituality
- I will be prettier and have an even more energetic personality (so more attractive in many ways)—Self Esteem
- I will have a better professional "look" to put out in the world —Work

As my client finished this exercise she had a remarkable revelation. She wrote, "this exercise has made me realize that my daily efforts and time commitments don't match my internal goals! I spend a lot of time working, but that's about it! WOW! That's bad!! And no wonder I'm stressed most days."

So, to all of you who are still relying on willpower to get you your desired results, I urge you to look to your values and link nutrition to the things that mean the most to you. This will give you the purpose, not will, to help you actualize all that you desire in your life.

clarified butter: ghee

Clarified butter or ghee has incredible healing and cooking properties and has been used in Ayurvedic traditions for over 5000 years. It has been incorporated into many of your nutritional lifestyles for its nourishing affects. Ghee is butter with the milk solids removed making for an excellent option for those with dairy sensitivities.

In *Healing with Whole Foods,* Paul Pitchford explains,

> Ghee enhances the ojas, an essence that governs the tissues
> of the body and balances the hormones. Ample ojas ensures
> a strong mind and body, resistance against disease, and is
> essential for longevity.[1]

In India, it is a common practice to consume one tablespoon of ghee in the morning to maintain alertness, mental acuity, to promote immunity and bowel regularity.

Clarified butter contains butyric acid, a fatty acid that has anti-aging, anticancer and antiviral properties. Butyric acid contains antioxidants that prevent free-radical damage, which may be why it has been found to be helpful in the prevention and treatment of cancer and Alzheimer's disease. According to Dr. Rudolph Ballentine, the author of *Radical Healing,* "in the presence of butyrates, malignant cells have become normal."[2] From an antiviral perspective, Ballentine explains,

> When incorporated into the cell membrane, butyric acid
> increases the human cell's production of the antiviral substance
> interferon by 25% and it inhibits the reproduction of viruses in
> the cells of tissue cultures.[3]

The butyric acid in ghee also has anti-inflammatory principles and has been used to promote the healing and rejuvenation of gastro-intestinal inflammations such as colitis and ulcers.

Adding one teaspoon of ghee at a meal will increase "agni" (digestive fire), which will help improve the breakdown, assimilation and absorption of foods. This is especially beneficial for vata types, who tend to have low digestive fire (see Tip 46). Adding an essential fat such as ghee to steamed vegetables will also help maximize the absorption of the fat-soluble nutrients found in the vegetables. In *Diet and Nutrition: A Holistic Approach,* Dr. Rudolph Ballentine states "ghee will magnify the nutritional value of its con-stituents."[4] This is why in Ayurvedic healing and cooking, ghee is combined with spices and herbs, so when ingested the medicinal effects of the seasonings are maximized.

Ghee is ideal for frying or sautéing, adding to steamed vegetables, as a spread, or stirring it into rice or other whole grain dishes. In any recipe, you can likely use ghee in place of butter or oil. Ghee can also be found in Indian grocery stores or spice stores and at some Superstore locations in the ethnic foods section. You can also make your own ghee.

ghee
2 lbs organic unsalted butter

1 Heat 2 lbs of organic unsalted butter in a saucepan until it boils.
2 Lower the heat to maintain a light, rolling boil.
3 When foam at the top begins to condense and thicken, it should be skimmed off.
4 After 12–15 minutes (or once the liquid is evaporated), when boiling stops and a frying-oil sound begins, quickly remove from heat and allow to cool for 1–2 minutes.

5   Pour the clarified butter into earthenware or a glass jar or
    bowl. The sediment at the bottom of the pot and the skimming
    from the top are milk solids that can be discarded, or used on
    vegetables. Makes 1 lb of ghee.

Ghee can be kept in the refrigerator indefinitely, but can also be
stored at room temperature for several weeks.

It is important to note that even though you are boiling and heating the butter, the nutrient value does not change.

Using ghee is a fabulous way to add variety and flavour to your
meals. Clarified butter is delicious! So spread your wings, stimulate your taste buds, be adventurous and try something new.

kitcheri recipe

"A man may esteem himself happy when that which is his food is also his medicine." –Henry David Thoreau

This East Indian meal is very easy to digest and can be eaten all year long. It has a perfect combination of protein, essential fats and carbohydrates, so you could live on it for quite some time if need be. It is especially recommended for anyone with digestive difficulties, malabsorption of food, chronic fatigue, loss of appetite, post-partum, detoxification or if feeling under the weather with a stomach flu or cold. This concoction makes a great medicine to rebuild the body and is ideal for all Ayurvedic doshas.

kitcheri[1]

1 cup split yellow mung beans
2 cups basmati rice
1 inch fresh ginger root, peeled and chopped
1 small handful fresh cilantro leaves, chopped
2 tbsp ghee
1 tsp turmeric
1 tsp coriander powder
1 tsp cumin powder
1 tsp whole cumin seeds
1 tsp mustard seeds
1 tsp kosher salt
1 pinch hing (asafoetida)—optional (found in Indian grocery stores)
7–10 cups water

1 Wash beans and rice together until water runs clear.
2 In a large pot on medium heat mix ginger, ghee, turmeric, coriander powder, cumin powder, cumin seeds, mustard seeds, salt and hing and stir together for a few minutes.

3 Add rice and beans and stir again. Add water and salt and bring to a boil. Boil for 10 minutes. You can also add vegetables to the pot if you so desire.

4 Turn heat to low, cover pot and continue to cook until rice and beans become soft (about 30–40 minutes).

5 Add the cilantro leaves just before serving.

Stuffing is always a holiday favorite and a match made in heaven for that big, juicy turkey. This year, try a healthy alternative to your stuffing so you can enjoy and indulge without the guilt or the bloat! If you are following a gluten-free, yeast-free, grain-free and low carbohydrate nutritional lifestyle, this stuffing recipe is an excellent alternative.

vegetable chestnut stuffing[1]

1 tbsp coconut oil, butter or ghee
5 med garlic cloves, minced
2 large onions, chopped
8 large stalks celery, chopped
2 med carrots, coarsely shredded
2 med kohlrabi, peeled and chopped
2 med apples, finely chopped
3 cups chopped Italian flat-leaf parsley, packed
2 cups coarsely chopped chestnuts or sliced water chestnuts
1 tbsp black currants
1 tbsp thyme, 2 tsp sage, ½ tsp rosemary or
2 tbsp poultry seasoning
1 tsp sea salt
½ tsp freshly ground pepper

1   In large pot, melt oil or butter. Add minced garlic and
    onions and sauté until vegetables are translucent.
    Add celery, carrots, kohlrabi and apple and sauté until
    vegetables start to soften. Remove from heat.
2   Add chopped parsley, chestnuts, currants, herbs and salt
    and pepper. Mix together well.
3   Stuff turkey.

4   When turkey is done, scoop out stuffing and put into
    serving bowl. Cover until it's time to eat.

To complement your delicious turkey and stuffing, enjoy this great natural cranberry sauce recipe from the kitchen of Community Natural Foods. This is a much healthier alternative to opening up a can of cranberry sauce that is full of preservatives and high-fructose corn syrup.

cranberry sauce

1 lb fresh or frozen organic cranberries
1 ½ cups unpasteurized honey
½ cup water
½ cup fresh squeezed orange juice
2 tbsp grated orange zest

1   Combine ingredients in a large pot.
2   Cook uncovered over medium heat until the
    cranberries pop open and the mixture thickens (10 or
    more minutes).
3   Let cool and refrigerate.
4   Serve cold with your delicious free-range, organic turkey.

And… if you must dabble in the chocolate for dessert, choose organic dark chocolate. It is made of pure cocoa and no white sugar or other sweeteners added. The antioxidant content is actually higher than drinking a glass of red wine! Also choose high quality chocolates such as Bernard Callebaut and Godiva. These chocolates are made with pure ingredients, have no additives, preservatives, food dyes, palm kernel oil or high-fructose corn syrup.
    Here's to healthy holiday eating! Enjoy!

"Eat the way nature intended." –John Douillard

The time of summer days lasting longer than summer nights has come to its end. Welcome to the season of the harvest.

Autumn is the time for personal reflection or turning within, moving away from summer—the time of being outward, social, energetic and in tune with nature. It is a good time for writing, work, family, home projects and doing activities that make you content (painting, knitting, reading, etc.). The busy whimsical summer is fading and the grounding and balanced routine is emphasized.

Autumn is also the time to move away from summer's higher carbohydrate diet that was filled with plentiful fruits, colorful salads and lighter lower fat proteins like fish, yogurt and skinless chicken and turkey breasts. It is the time to move toward a higher protein diet, to reduce fruit consumption and begin eating more steamed and cooked vegetables than raw ones. Pumpkin and squash soups, roasted root vegetables and lamb, brown rice with almonds and buffalo meat sauce over spaghetti squash are excellent fall dishes.

As John Douillard explains in *The 3-Season Diet,* "the fall harvest is the time to gather the last growths of vegetation, along with nuts and whole grains that will see us through the long winter months."[1] Naturally, this is when grapes are harvested to make wine, when people clear the last of their gardens and preserve, and farmers gather hay into barns.

The fall harvest is the season to begin to consume higher purine proteins including dark poultry, wild game and lamb. Dairy products such as cottage cheese are also recommended at this time of year. More essential fats such as ghee, olive, coconut, sesame, sunflower and cod liver oils will help lubricate our skin and mucous membranes and keep us warm and insulated for the colder months to come. The most balancing whole grains for this season are brown rice, amaranth, quinoa and oats. Nuts and seeds are all good, paying particular attention to sunflower seeds and walnuts. The best beans to eat are mung. Autumn fruits include apples, pears, grapes, tomatoes, avocado, oranges, lemons, lime and grapefruit. Root vegetables are in abundance such as squash, pumpkin, carrots, beets, turnip and parsnip, but other fibrous vegetables such as Brussels sprouts, artichokes, seaweed, spinach and fennel are also welcomed.

It is important to note that if you need to avoid high glycemic or starchy foods it is best to follow the following nutrition tidbits. Avoid the root vegetables that leave no color on your cutting board when you cut into them (parsnips, turnips, white potatoes and corn). The colorful root vegetables such as carrots, squash, beets and pumpkin would be more ideal. You can also control your blood sugar levels by eating root vegetables with protein and a leafy green. Never eat root vegetables with another starch such as a whole grain.

Colds and flu are common in fall, but can be prevented by eating seasonal foods and adding hot spices, ginger, chilis, garlic and onions regularly to the diet. All these foods help reduce and clear out excess mucous in the body. Burdock and comfrey are also excellent herbs to use for this purpose. Regular nasal douches with a Neti-Pot (sold at the Hoffman Centre for Integrative Medicine and some health food stores) are also recommended.

Tone up your exercise program with weights or yoga. Daily exercise will help regulate your weight and prevent the tendency to gain a few pounds through the fall and winter months. Weight training will turn those natural few added pounds into muscle as opposed to fat. Weights and yoga are also very grounding exercises that suit the energy of fall, as leaves, apples and the sun all move toward the earth.

Autumn is the time for inner reflection, an excellent time to make meditation a regular part of your daily lifestyle, if it is not already. Deep breathing is also an excellent way to keep the lungs and nasal passageways clear so excess mucous does not build up.

Eating seasonally plays a significant role in maintaining balance and wellness throughout the year. To all my readers, have a refreshing season. Welcome the crisp air, embrace the red, orange and yellow leaves, admire the harvest moon and enjoy incorporating the wonderful tastes and textures of the fall harvest.

"When we fill ourselves with a soup as delicious as a consommé, it delights our bodies, and yet more our souls."
–Paul Scarron

The following are some delicious and seasonal soups that will keep you warm on a cool fall evening. Enjoy these soups as a perfect complement to any protein you desire.

carrot ginger soup[1]

1 tbsp ghee, coconut oil or olive oil
2 onions, coarsely chopped
1 red pepper, chopped
2 cloves garlic
9 large carrots, cut in chunks
1 large potato, peeled, cut in chunks
4 cups organic vegetable broth
2 tbsp fresh dill
½–1 cup coconut milk (for thicker soup) or water
1 tsp ginger, grated

1 In saucepan, heat oil on medium heat.
2 Add onions and red pepper, sauté until golden. Add garlic and sauté 2–3 minutes. If necessary add a little water to prevent burning.
3 Add carrots, potato and broth.
4 Bring to a boil. Reduce heat and simmer covered for 25–30 minutes, stirring occasionally.
5 Purée soup. Add dill, salt and pepper to taste. Blend in coconut milk or water and fresh ginger.

fresh asparagus soup[2]

1 ½ lbs fresh asparagus
1 tbsp coconut oil or ghee
1 large onion, chopped
1 stalk celery, chopped
3 ½ cups organic chicken broth
1 potato, peeled and diced
1 cup organic plain yogurt
2 tbsp basil leaves

1   Cut off and reserve about 24 asparagus tips.
2   Chop remaining asparagus into small pieces.
3   In large saucepan, over medium heat, heat oil. Add onion and
    celery; cook, stirring often, until softened.
4   Add chicken broth, chopped asparagus and potato. Bring to a
    boil, reduce heat, cover and simmer for 15 minutes.
5   Purée until smooth in blender or food processor.
6   Return soup to saucepan. Heat until very hot.
7   Whisk yogurt until smooth; stir into soup.
8   Steam reserved asparagus tips until tender crisp. Scatter on top
    of each serving and sprinkle with fresh basil.

roasted butternut squash and apple soup[3]

½ butternut squash, peeled and coarsely diced
2 tbsp coconut oil or ghee
1 yellow onion, diced
1 tbsp dried or fresh thyme
1 Granny smith apple, peeled and coarsely diced
1 cup organic vegetable or chicken stock
1 cup water
½ tsp Celtic sea salt and pepper to taste

1   Preheat oven to 450˚F.
2   Put the squash and 1 tbsp oil or ghee in a bowl and stir well, making sure to coat the squash thoroughly.
3   Spoon the squash onto a cookie sheet and bake for 15–20 minutes, or until the edges are slightly brown. Remove from the oven and allow to cool slightly.
4   In a pot, heat 1 tbsp oil and add onion and quickly sauté for 2–4 minutes.
5   Add thyme, squash, apple, stock and water. Bring to a boil and cook until the squash and apple are soft, about 15 minutes. Remove from heat.
6   Purée with a blender or food processor until smooth. Add salt and pepper to taste.

curried zucchini soup[4]

1 tsp ghee, coconut oil or olive oil
1 tsp curry powder
½ tsp ground cumin
½ tsp garlic powder
Pinch of red pepper flakes
1 cup yellow onion, coarsely diced
2 zucchini coarsely diced
1 cup organic vegetable broth
1 cup water
1 tbsp raisins
1 tbsp dried cranberries
½ tsp Celtic sea salt

1   In a pot over medium heat, add oil, curry, cumin, garlic, red pepper and onion. Mix well, turn the heat to low and cover.
2   Cook for 5 minutes or until onions are translucent.

3 Add the zucchini, stock and water. Increase the heat to medium–high and boil, uncovered, until zucchini is soft, about 10 minutes. Cover, remove pot from heat and let stand for at least 5 minutes.

4 Purée with a food processor or blender until smooth. Add the raisins, cranberries, salt and pepper and blend again.

protein shakes

Getting tired of the same old protein shake morning after morning? The following are some ideas to add some variety and flavor to your nutritious morning regimen.

- Switch up your protein powders. If you have been using the same one, try using a high quality whey, hemp protein, rice protein or goat whey, which are all available at the Hoffman Centre for Integrative Medicine and health food stores.
- Try using different kinds of berries. Blueberries tend to make a shake thin and watery so try raspberries and strawberries for a thicker shake. Or, because blueberries are high in anti-oxidants, combine 25% blueberries and 75% other berries.
- In my opinion, a banana makes or breaks a shake—so add a fresh or frozen banana to your shake. If you use frozen bananas, remove the peel before you freeze the bananas. If you don't like bananas, try papaya, mango or peaches.
- Add healthy fats to your shake. If you use flavored fish oils, try a new flavor (peach, orange or lemon). If you want to try another type of oil that is high in omega-3, use hemp or mac-adamia nut oil for a more nutty taste. A little sesame oil can also be used for a slight spicy flavor.
- At least one teaspoon of cinnamon powder always brings great flavor to a shake. Cinnamon is also excellent for con-trolling and balancing blood sugar levels—ideal if you are using higher glycemic fruits.
- Vanilla powder or extract can also be used for a nice taste and aromatic touch to your shake.
- Cardamom powder can also be used for more flavor and is a nice warming touch in the fall and winter.

- Alternative milks such as rice, soy or almond are not recommended as they are processed and high in sugar. It is best to thicken your shake with coconut milk or plain organic yogurt.
- A couple of tablespoons of coconut oil can be added if you are in need of a lot of energy (athletes, healing from cancer/chemotherapy, low thyroid function, during pregnancy and post-partum). Coconut oil is also beneficial for people with gut dysbiosis, or who are in need of losing weight.
- Finely grated organic lemon, lime, orange or grapefruit peel also enhances the flavor in a shake and makes the shake smell great. These peels also contain potent anti-oxidants (phytochemicals), so they can boost the effects of your shake even more.
- A bit of 100% almond butter, hazelnut or other nut butter can thicken the shake and add a nutty flavor.
- For the kids or for a treat for yourself, add some pure cocoa powder for a chocolate-y flavor.
- If you ever need to sweeten your shake, you can always add a drop of Stevia. Be careful with the Stevia powder as the line between pleasantly sweet and an awful aftertaste is thin.

Protein shakes are healthy, fast and convenient. They provide a perfect balance of macronutrients. They are also a great way to boost nutrient intake. So, don't leave your shake behind because you are getting bored. Instead, give your shake a boost to enhance flavor and re-stimulate your senses.

For a real change, try these two quick, healthy breakfast drinks:

nut shake[1]

1 tbsp raw nut butter (almond, macadamia, walnut, pecan etc.)
1 tbsp dry, unsweetened coconut

2 cups clean, filtered water

1 whole organic egg

1 tsp Stevia

1 Blend all of the ingredients in a blender, except egg, until smooth and frothy.
2 Add whole egg and pulse only briefly to blend.
3 Pour into glass and enjoy.

sunny almond shake[2]

2 tbsp organic almonds

2 tbsp organic sunflower seeds

2 tbsp organic flax seeds

3 cups clean, filtered water (1–1 ½ cups if using juice)

½ cup fresh apple cider or pineapple juice

½ cup raspberries or blueberries

½ tsp vanilla extract

½ tsp nutmeg

1 Process almonds, sunflower and flax seeds in covered blender, until coarsely ground.
2 Pour in water slowly at first, letting blades reduce ingredients to a thick consistency. Add remaining liquid and blend.
3 Add juice, berries, vanilla extract and nutmeg, and blend until frothy. Pour in glass and drink immediately.

Sodium has become nutritionally misunderstood, yet it is one of the most important minerals the body needs to maintain homeostasis and function optimally. We have had such fear about ingesting sodium, that we may have actually starved our bodies of a significant nutrient and as a result, may have caused an imbalance in the body. According to Dr. Bernard Jensen, "the world at large is suffering from diseases caused by sodium hunger."[1]

The functions of sodium in the body are numerous and extensive. Sodium is abundantly stored in the stomach and joints, so if you experience any symptoms in those areas of the body (heartburn, ulcers, joint pain, etc.), you may be sodium deficient. Sodium keeps joints and ligaments supple (important for those with arthritis) and feeds the friendly bacteria in the bowel.

One of the most significant effects of sodium on our health is its power to create alkalinity and neutralize acids in the body.

In *The Chemistry of Man,* Dr. Bernard Jensen writes,

> If it wasn't for the neutralizing power of sodium in the walls of
> the stomach and bowel, they would be eaten away by the pow-
> erful acids, enzymes and digestive juices secreted as foods
> are eaten."[2]

For those who work out, sodium is important to neutralize the lactic acid created during anaerobic activity.

Sodium keeps calcium in solution in the blood and sodium in the blood helps regulate the fluid balance in the body. The nerves use sodium and potassium to relay electrical nerve impulses throughout the body. The balance of sodium and potassium is also necessary to flush heavy metals out of the cells—which is why many of you seeing Dr. Hoffman and going through a detoxification protocol are taking Selectrolytes—a unique balanced formula of electrolytes. Taking Selectrolytes also ensures you are hydrating your body intracellularly.

The confusion about sodium comes when it is ingested from the wrong sources. Common table salt contains inorganic sodium whereas fruits, vegetables and other whole foods such as whey, egg yolks and fish contain an organic form of sodium which the body recognizes and utilizes for many biochemical processes, as listed above. According to Dr. Jensen, it is the inorganic sodium found in table salt as well as in most processed, manufactured, packaged and canned foods that are unhealthy to the human body. Refined table salt is dried at over 1,200 degrees Fahrenheit, which destroys all its essential minerals. This temperature also changes the chemical structure of the salt. Conventional processing also adds harmful additives and chemicals to whiten the salt to make it look "pure" as well as to make it sift easily through saltshakers. It is this form of sodium that if eaten in excess, can become detrimental to our health and contribute to specific conditions such as hypertension and fluid retention.

What about kosher salt? Although kosher salt usually has no additives and is less salty than table salt, it still inorganic sodium, as is iodinized salt. The large crystals of kosher salt absorb more moisture than other forms of salt, and this makes kosher salt excellent for curing meats. That is essentially where the name comes from. The salt itself is not kosher meaning it doesn't conform to Jewish food laws, but this salt is used to make meat kosher. The Jewish Holy Book (the Torah) prohibits consumption of any blood and a common way of removing the final traces of blood from meat is to soak and salt it.

I always speak of biochemical individuality, and the concept is relevant to your salt intake as well. The best way to determine if you need to boost or limit your sodium intake in your diet is to look at your fasting chemistry profile which shows the serum sodium level. You can ask to have this profile done by Dr. Hoffman or your family physician. The sodium level should be 139—an ideal range is 136 to 142. If it is much lower, you probably need more sodium; if it is higher, you probably want to restrict salt intake.

If you are going to use salt, only use and purchase natural Celtic Sea Salt from the health food stores. It is not heated, processed, altered or contaminated with chemicals. In fact, Celtic Sea Salt actually has a grey color to it, meaning that it is rich in minerals, quite a difference from your typical table salt which is void of all essential minerals. Use sea salt in moderation.

The best place to get your sodium is from whole foods. Sodium is found naturally in many foods. It is especially abundant in powdered goat or cow's whey, dulse and kelp (seaweeds), celery, kale, asparagus, leafy greens, okra, parsley, beets, black mission figs, chickpeas and liquid chlorophyll. If you ingest enough of these foods, then adding Celtic Sea Salt is likely not necessary. If you do like to salt your foods, you can also purchase powdered seaweeds (kelp or dulse) at a health food store and use it as a replacement in your saltshaker. This is an excellent way to add a natural salt taste to your meals and seaweed is also rich in iodine which is excellent for those who need thyroid support, it also aids in digestion and is an incredible cancer fighter. Sheets of seaweed can also be used to flavor soups or stir-fry instead of flavoring them with harmful table salt.

It is important to note that those with hypertension, renal failure, congestive heart failure, excess weight, water retention or a kapha body type, should avoid using any type of salt.

Give your body a boost of organic sodium and try Veal Joint Broth from *Sally Fallon's Nourishing Traditions.* This natural source of sodium is great for the glands, stomach, ligaments and digestive disorders, as well as helping to retain youth in the body.

veal joint broth[3]

1 clean fresh uncut veal joint
1 small stalk celery, finely cut
1 1/2 cups apple peelings, finely cut
2 cups potato peelings, finely cut
1/2 cup chopped parsley, finely cut
2 beets, grated
1 large parsnip, finely cut
1 onion, finely cut
1/2 cup okra, finely cut or 1 tsp powdered okra (if you can't find it fresh)

1   Wash veal in cold water, put into a large cooking pot; cover half with water.
2   Add vegetables and greens.
3   Simmer all ingredients for 4–5 hours; strain off liquid and discard solid ingredients.
4   There should be about 1 ½ quarts of liquid. Drink hot or warm. Keep refrigerated.

"Other than the oxygen you inhale, the only other source of healthy input for your body comes from what you eat and drink."
–from *Spa Medicine*

It's a delight to find such a powerful nutritive to add so effortlessly to nutritional lifestyles. Chlorophyll, also known as, "green magic," "concentrated sun power," and "the blood of plant life," is the basis of all plant life. Chlorophyll resembles the red content of human blood, and the life force and magnetism it gives to plants is beneficial for us as well.

Here are some of the many reasons you may want to include chlorophyll as part of your regular nutritional lifestyle:

- High in oxygen—the cells of the body and the brain function at an optimal level in a highly oxygenated environment
- Oxygenation increases energy, stamina and physical and mental performance
- Antibacterial properties prevent the growth and development of harmful bacteria
- Increases the function of the heart and the lungs—helpful for asthma
- Promotes bowel regularity and cleanses the colon
- Prevents tooth decay
- Heals the stomach lining and is effective for ulcers
- Controls blood sugars—beneficial for hypoglycemia, insulin resistance or Type II diabetes
- Combats the hardening of arteries
- Tissue builder—great for recovery after surgery or exercising
- Raises iron in the blood—good for anemia
- Antioxidant properties inhibit the action of carcinogens and may help prevent cancer

- Helps purify the liver and gets bile moving regularly
- Improves hepatitis
- Regulates menstruation and can be used to fight vaginitis or candidiasis
- Aids in detoxification and removing heavy metals from the body
- Eliminates body odors
- Eliminates bad breath
- Its high alkalinity helps neutralize acidity in the body
- Reduces inflammation making it beneficial for colitis, arthritis, sinusitis, psoriasis and eczema
- High in magnesium which will help control and regulate calcium levels in the blood

You can purchase liquid chlorophyll at health food stores. I recommend the Nature's Way product. Add a tablespoon of liquid chlorophyll in a glass of filtered water twice a day and enjoy the fantastic health benefits as well as a fresh mint taste in your water. You can also stop at any juice bar and grab a shot of organically grown wheatgrass, which contains 70% chlorophyll.

Biorhythmically, as the seasons change so too can the shape of our bodies. Some researchers call this the "hibernation theory." They say it is in our genetic code to gain weight during the winter months and shed it during spring and summer. After all, cave men and women didn't have central heating. They probably packed on a few extra pounds of insulation each year to make it through the cold winter months. It seems that as the weather gets colder, the body naturally gains an average of 5–7 lbs to conserve energy and insulate itself. Plain and simple, fat insulates and the fatter we are, the warmer we are.

While it may be the body's innate wisdom to pack on a few extra pounds during the fall and winter months, other factors can contribute to seasonal weight gain that can take you above and beyond what is natural and healthy. Unless those extra pounds are controlled, combatted and shed each spring, they just stay in bigger numbers year after year, contributing to health problems such as obesity, diabetes, high blood pressure and heart disease. Here are some tips to help you battle the bulge through the winter season:

Cold and or stormy weather makes it difficult to exercise outdoors. On some days, even braving the elements to drive to the gym seems like too much effort. But exercise is crucial to avoid weight gain in the winter. So set a regular yet varied fitness schedule including both cardio and strength training. If you are unmotivated, find a workout buddy with whom you'll meet. This will make a big difference in how often you show up at the gym. Pre-pay a personal trainer to motivate you and make you accountable.

Maintain your water intake. We tend to drink less water in the cold weather, but because it is so dry in Calgary, our need for water increases. Hydrate your cells and skin with room temperature filtered water.

Get as much natural sunlight as you can. Diminished sunlight and vitamin D in winter reduces the brain's production of serotonin, the mood-boosting chemical that helps suppress overeating and food cravings for high calorie, fat-producing carbohydrates such as cakes, cookies, ice cream and chips. Try to spend at least 30 minutes outdoors each day, ideally during the brightest part of the day. Bundle up and take a walk outside at lunchtime, or go hiking, skiing or ice skating on the weekend. Take cod liver oil for excellent essential fats and vitamin D.

Shorter days and longer nights may induce feelings of depression, fatigue and cravings for sweets and starches. One of the easiest and best ways to curb cravings in winter is to increase your protein and essential fatty acid intake, which we naturally tend to do anyway at this time of year. Approximately 20 extra grams of protein daily is needed (i.e. ¾ cup cottage cheese, two eggs and a slice of mozzarella cheese,one cup of lentils or kidney beans, ½ can wild salmon). Adding more essential fats will also help reduce cravings. A little extra olive oil, ghee or coconut oil is often all it takes to prevent sugar cravings.

L-tryptophan is an amino acid and natural winter mood-booster which can be found in turkey, cottage cheese, roasted pumpkin seeds, baked potatoes with their skins on and kelp. To make serotonin, the body also needs a good supply of vitamin B6 which is found in carrots, fish, lentils, peas, potato, spinach and sunflower seeds. So it is a good idea to increase your dietary intake of all of these foods during the colder months.

Another factor that contributes to those extra pounds is constant indulgences throughout the holiday season. From October to February there are continual sugar-filled and food-oriented holidays such as Thanksgiving, Halloween, Chanukah, Christmas, New

Year's Eve, Super Bowl and Valentines Day. On average, our sugar and alcohol consumption is much higher in the winter months than it is in spring and summer—which most definitely contributes to weight gain.

You don't want to avoid the holiday gatherings but you can do a few things to prevent indulging excessively. First, never go to a party hungry! Eat something one or two hours BEFORE you go, maybe a colorful salad with some tuna, chicken or turkey, hard boiled eggs, organic yogurt or a handful of nuts with a piece of fruit. This will suppress hunger and not leave much room for overeating.

So much of our eating is not related to hunger. The more variety of foods at an event, the more likely we are to eat more food. The best thing you can do at a buffet is ASSESS the situation, as opposed to ATTACK the situation! Walk through first and take note of all the foods that are there. Decide what you would like to have, what would be the healthiest and what you know you should avoid, and then build your plate. Eat slowly so you become satiated before you get up for seconds. It is fascinating that when more people are around we feel we have to load our plate up or go for seconds before we are finished what we have, because we think there won't be enough food! Don't be a vulture because really, how many times have you gone to a dinner party where there has been a shortage of food? There are always leftovers.

Leftovers are another way to pack on excess weight. Send your company home with the leftovers, especially the desserts. If they remain in your house, you will inevitably eat them. Bring extra Halloween candy and other tempting foods to shelters or families who may not have had the opportunity to indulge.

Remember to have fun! When you go out and celebrate all the upcoming holidays and festivities, it should be a people event that just happens to involve food, not a food event that just happens to involve people!

Finally, enjoy fall and winter and welcome those few extra natural and healthy pounds for warmth, conservation and insulation. By following the tips above, you will prevent gaining any more weight your body needs or desires and successfully battle the seasonal bulge.

In Ayurveda, food is categorized into six tastes (known as rasas): sweet, sour, salty, pungent, bitter and astringent.

- Sweet: Ghee, meat, honey, rice, banana, coconut, raisins
- Sour: Yogurt, cheese, vinegar, grapes, citrus fruits, tomato
- Salty: Celtic sea salt, seaweed, olives, salted nuts
- Pungent: Chili peppers, black pepper, hot spices, garlic, onions
- Bitter: Spinach, kale and other dark leafy greens
- Astringent: Unripe fruit, beans, cranberries, pomegranate and black tea

According to Ayurvedic medicine, the body is made up of different elements. Based on those elements, specific tastes are needed to create balance and satiation at every meal.

The immediate experience of these tastes, affects your Ayurvedic body type (dosha). Some tastes balance your dosha while others can create an imbalance. For example, a pitta type, made up of the elements fire and water, does very well with bitter tastes; the bitterness cools pitta's fire and has a drying effect on the water element. If a pitta type eats too many pungent (hot, spicy) foods, the fiery pitta body can heat up too much—causing aggravation, imbalance and conditions associated with excess heat.

Both physiologically and psychologically, different body types respond differently to the six tastes. Flavoring, spicing and combining tastes at every meal then becomes a science and something necessary to understand and consider as part of your nutritional lifestyle, in order to maintain balance in the body.

To make it simple, you can create your own personal spice blend based on your unique body type or dosha (vata, pitta and kapha). These blends can be added to your meals to help you ensure that you are receiving the right balance of tastes for your individual body type. The following are the 3 spice blends recommended for each dosha:

- Vata Spice favors sweet, sour and salt tastes: cardamom, cumin, ginger, cinnamon, nutmeg, asafetida and salt
- Pitta Spice favors sweet, bitter and astringent tastes: cumin, coriander, fennel, turmeric, stevia and salt
- Kapha Spice favors pungent, bitter and astringent tastes: coriander, ginger, mustard, turmeric, cinnamon and cayenne

It is ideal to purchase these spices in bulk and create and compile your own personalized spice mix. Put the concoction in a saltshaker and add it to all of your foods. Sprinkle it on salads, steamed vegetables, soups, over eggs, meats, stews, chili, etc. The possibilities are endless and the balancing effects are essential for wellness.

Balancing your Ayurvedic dosha is a key piece to nutritional mastery. Step Four of the 7 Step program will help you to determine your Ayurvedic dosha, learn how to balance your foods and ensure ongoing balance. If you do not have the opportunity to work with me, you can also read *Perfect Health* by Deepak Chopra to determine your unique body type.

If you ever wonder about the purpose in maintaining your optimum nutritional lifestyle, or question why you work so hard to stick to your diet when most people around you seem indifferent to what they put into their mouths, I offer you a brief yet profound message with this nutritional tip.

> It's of value to think of health as that condition of the individual that makes possible the highest enjoyment of life. Health, when thought of simply as the absence of disease, is a standard of mediocrity, but when thought of as a quality of life it is a standard of inspiration and ever-increasing achievement.
> –Jesse Williams

Sound nutrition is the vehicle that can lead your body to a state of optimum wellness. An optimum nutritional lifestyle will take you above and beyond "a standard of mediocrity." It will separate you from the masses, help you actualize your full potential and make you grateful for every day you wake up with energy, clarity and well being.

So don't doubt your nutrition. Know with certainty nutrition is serving a purpose—to help you master all that you desire in life.

"Health is a personal responsibility, and a person can accomplish nothing without full commitment." –Dr. Roger Rogers

Optimum wellness through sound nutrition cannot and never will be found in a pill. I believe it is the one thing that we will have to actualize for ourselves without the help of pharmaceuticals, technology or convenience food. And so it takes effort, commitment, time and purpose.

We are so used to a "quick fix" for everything and in many cases we get what we want with little effort. Perhaps this is why beginning to implement your sound nutritional lifestyle can feel overwhelming. It takes more advance thinking, time and effort to shop and cook this way. It can be a bit daunting when the reality sets in that no one can do this for you.

In these moments, realize that the journey is not about perfection. It is not about having to implement every nutritional recommendation I give you in the first month or even the first six months.

Recently, a client who'd first worked with me well over a year ago returned for a visit. "Sometimes," she said, "the journey is difficult and overwhelming. At times, it seemed like too much, too fast, too soon—and perhaps the timing just wasn't right." But instead of giving up, she created and owned her own nutritional pace, her own time frame and ways of shopping, cooking and balancing, and it has worked beautifully. Over the course of one year she slowly integrated the recommendations and actualized a sound and balanced nutritional lifestyle. She did reach her weight loss goals and restore the integrity of her digestive system. Now she feels better, enjoys improved energy and vitality, and maintains her weight. Did this take some effort, commitment, time and purpose? Yes, but she did it, she did it her way, and she reaps the wellness benefits. Now she is ready to take the next step into understanding how to fuel her metabolic type.

So, forget perfectionism and focus on purpose! Take the pressure off of yourself while maintaining the effort and commitment. Set some realistic goals or time frames. Put the recommendations I created for you in Step Two on your fridge, computer or kitchen table and read them often until you remember how to do everything. Highlight the information most important to remember. Over the course of a few months explore different grocery stores, markets and health food stores and find one or two that you really enjoy. If life is just too overwhelming right now, just visualize the change, and you can commit to making the time for the change in lifestyle down the road, when you can see the clearing in the forest, so to speak.

Always remember that "wellness" medicine is about an equal working partnership between you and your wellness practitioner. Certainly it is not about the doctor giving you a pill to make it all better and it is not about disempowering you and putting control in a "healer's" hands to fix everything. It is about empowering yourself to be the healer within. So stay the course, don't fall for the fantasy "quick fix" because it does not exist when it comes to health. The only way to achieve wellness is through your own intention and action. It is your effort. It is your commitment. It is your time and life and purpose. So do it your way. There are no rules. It is your journey.

"Our lives are not in the lap of the gods, but in the lap of our cooks." –Lin Yutang

I invite you to all have dinner with me, non-locally of course! I would love to share with you one of my favorite meals. It comes directly from the heart and kitchen of my mom, who is an expert in what food is all about—cooking with love.

Though there are a few ingredients in these two recipes that you wouldn't use in the daily nutritional lifestyles I have created for you (brown sugar, Worcester sauce), and some steps may not be optimal (e.g., heating olive oil at high temperatures), I still rank this as a 95% healthy meal. It is particularly good for mixed and protein metabolic body types, a wonderful balancing meal for vata types and for everyone else, a perfect fall/winter seasonal dish. So what is it, you ask??? Butterfly Leg of Lamb served with Roasted Root Vegetables. My mouth is watering as I write! Delicious!!!

roasted root vegetables[1]

2 beets
4 parsnips
2 yams
1 turnip
4 carrots
2 red onions

marinade ingredients

1 garlic clove
1 tbsp balsamic vinegar
3 tbsp olive oil
2 tbsp brown sugar
1 tbsp thyme

Celtic Sea Salt and pepper to taste
1 tbsp rosemary

1 Peel and cut all vegetables into small cubes.
2 Put all marinade ingredients in a large bowl.
3 Put vegetables in the bowl and allow to sit in the marinade for a maximum of 2 hours.
4 Bake on a baking sheet at 500°F for 35–40 minutes.

butterfly leg of lamb

6–7lb leg of lamb
2 tbsp Worcester sauce
Mustard to taste
Homemade Italian salad dressing to taste

1 Coat leg of lamb with mustard, Worcester sauce and home-made Italian salad dressing. Allow to marinade overnight.
2 Roast the leg (fat side up), uncovered at 325°F for 3 hours. Baste the lamb a few times with the marinade.
3 Serve this delicious meal as is, or with a salad or steamed broccoli. Enjoy!!!

Note that, if you are Type II diabetic, insulin resistant, hypoglycemic, or trying to lose weight, and are concerned about eating the root vegetables, this recipe should be okay for you. Why? You are slowing the spike of blood sugars with a high purine protein such as lamb. Of course, always opt for a small serving of root vegetables and focus on a bigger portion of salad or broccoli. Remember the 95% rule! What you do most of the time is what counts.

"It is confidence in our bodies, minds and spirits that allows us to keep looking for new adventures, new directions to grow in, and new lessons to learn—which is what life is all about."
–Oprah Winfrey

Do you know anyone who thinks his or her own body is perfect? I don't. There is no question that there are things about our bodies that we like and dislike. What if we realized that the things we dislike about our bodies actually serve a purpose in our lives? What if we knew that what we love about our bodies have drawbacks to our lives? At a weekend Breakthrough Experience® with Dr. John Demartini (www.drdemartini.com), I realized this truth and would like to share with you some of my insights to help you, too, better understand benefits you might not otherwise see.

For every area that I disliked about my body, I asked myself, how is this trait (of my body) serving me in my life? How is it in fact a benefit to me? The theme that kept recurring is that everything I disliked was the motivating factor in helping me find the best products, the best solutions, the best wellness practitioners, the best fitness trainers and the latest cutting-edge research on alleviating or improving the perceived issue, problem or condition. In a deep moment of gratitude, I saw that my "dislikes" of my physical body were supporting my highest value, which is the quest for physical health and wellness. These "dislikes" dissolved as I saw how they were serving my life. I also realized that my physical body is the vehicle for me to fulfill my vocational mission in life, which is to inspire, educate and motivate people to realize the significant impact sound nutrition has on achieving optimum wellness.

In a moment of deep gratitude, I knew the magnificence and perfection of my creation. I thanked my creator for what my body is, as it is. Each of us is a perfect creation and to deny the perfect purpose of our physical form is to deny the Grand Organized Design from which we all come. Who are we without loving all that we are and all that we look like?

If I can help you realize this transformational truth then I will be living out part of my mission in life. When you realize it, you will be living out your own mission with more confidence and certainty for who you are and what you do. In Step Five of my 7 Steps to Sound Nutrition™ program, I take you through this process and help you love your body for what it is, as it is. You, too, can reach a point of such life-affirming gratitude for who you are as you are. Now that is living!

"There is no love sincerer than the love of food"
–George Bernard Shaw

When the snow has finally fallen it seems fitting to start up some hearty, heart-warming and delicious winter soups. Winter is the best time to put the soup pot or crock pot to work and warm, soothe and satiate your body, mind and spirit throughout the season. So, how about joining me in the kitchen (non-locally of course!)? Together we'll make up fresh batches of these wonderful soups.

curried celery soup[1]

2 tsp olive oil
1 onion, chopped
1 leek, sliced
5 ½ cups celery, chopped
1 tbsp med or hot curry powder
1 ½ cups unpeeled potato, diced
3 ¾ cups vegetable or chicken stock
1 bouquet garni
2 tbsp chopped fresh mixed herbs
Salt to taste
Celery seeds and leaves, to garnish

1. Heat oil in large saucepan. Add the onion, leek and celery, cover and cook slowly for about 10 minutes, stirring occasionally.
2. Add the curry powder and continue cooking for 2 minutes, stirring occasionally.
3. Add the potatoes, stock and bouquet garni, cover and bring to a boil. Simmer for 20 minutes, until the vegetables are tender, but not too soft.

4   Remove and discard the bouquet garni. Set aside the soup to cool slightly before it is processed.

5   Transfer the soup to a blender or food processor and process in batches until smooth.

6   Add the mixed herbs, season to taste with salt and briefly process again. Return to saucepan and reheat slowly until hot. Ladle into bowls and garnish with celery seeds and celery leaves.

spiced lentil soup[2]

2 onions, minced

2 garlic cloves, crushed

4 tomatoes, roughly chopped

½ tsp turmeric

1 tsp ground cumin

6 cardamom pods

½ cinnamon stick

1 ⅓ cups red lentils, rinsed and drained

3 ½ cups water

14-oz can coconut milk

1 tbsp lime juice

Salt and pepper to taste

Cumin seeds, to garnish

1   Put the onions, garlic, tomatoes, turmeric, cumin, cardamom pods, cinnamon, lentils and water into a pot and bring to a boil. Lower the heat, cover and simmer for 20 minutes, or until lentils are soft.

2   Remove the cardamom pods and cinnamon stick. Purée the mixture in a blender or food processor. Press the soup through a strainer into the rinsed pot.

3   Reserve a bit of the coconut milk for garnish and add the remainder to the pot with the lime juice. Stir well and season with salt and pepper.

4   Reheat the soup slowly without boiling. Swirl in the reserved coconut milk and garnish with cumin seeds.

beet and lima bean soup[3]

2 tbsp olive oil

1 onion, sliced

1 tsp caraway seeds

Finely grated rind of ½ an organic orange

2 generous cups grated cooked beets

1 ½ cup beef broth

14-oz can lima beans, drained and rinsed

1 tbsp wine vinegar

4 tbsp sour cream (1 tbsp per bowl)—optional

4 tbsp chopped parsley, to garnish

1   Heat oil in large pot. Add onion, caraway seeds and orange peel and cook until soft but not colored.

2   Add beets, stock, lima beans and vinegar and simmer over low heat for 10 minutes.

3   Serve with sour cream and parsley.

lamb and lentil soup[4]

1 ½ quarts water or stock

2 pounds neck of lamb, cut into chops

½ onion chopped

1 garlic clove, crushed

1 bay leaf

1 clove

2 sprigs fresh thyme

1 ½ cups potatoes, cut into 1 inch pieces
½ cup red lentils
Salt and pepper
Fresh parsley, chopped

1   Put 1 ½ cups stock and meat in large pot with the onion, garlic,
    bay leaf, clove and sprigs of thyme and bring to a boil. Simmer
    for 1 hour until lamb is tender.
2   Add potato pieces and lentils to pot and season soup with salt
    and ground pepper. Add remaining stock or water to come just
    above the surface of the meat and vegetables; you may need
    more if soup becomes too thick during cooking.
3   Cover and allow to simmer for 25 minutes, or until the lentils are
    fully cooked.
4   Stir in parsley and serve.

We are familiar with "diet mentality." It goes like this: try a new diet program, see how long we can last, get some results, feel good for awhile, start getting bored, revert back to old eating patterns, give up and then (usually months later) try something new. Diet mentality is over, my friends. Sound nutrition is not about that. Sound nutrition is about creating a lifestyle that you can maintain indefinitely. It is about understanding, knowing and learning to connect with your body so intuitively that you just know exactly what foods and ratios of macronutrients will create balance and optimum wellness in your unique body type, and which ones will get in your way.

This doesn't happen in a single nutrition session. The Nutritional Assessment and Recommendations I customize for you in Step Two are initial steps on your journey to a state of optimum wellness. There is no question that with each step you will feel better, maximize your energy, trigger weight loss, change your cellular health, improve the integrity of your digestive system and alleviate symptoms, but your nutrition does not end there. It is just beginning. The initial steps you take create the foundation for wellness. Now you can advance to increasing states of wellness by learning and applying nutritional truths such as metabolic typing, Ayurvedic nutrition, seasonal eating and soulful nourishment—the very steps that teach you about the essence of who you are, how your body functions and how to feed that body accordingly.

I always talk about the importance of seasonal eating because it serves you and me so well! Quite simply, if you change your diet with the seasons, you will maintain balance and optimum wellness throughout the year. Those of you who are still eating summer diets in fall and winter might notice some unfavorable changes—you're not satiated, you experience food cravings again, you feel cold all the time, lack energy and already may have caught cold or flu. Those who still eat their winter diets in the spring, keep on the 5 pounds of natural winter weight, hold on to toxins and generally feel sluggish going into the summer months. Check in on your nutrition as each season changes. Come for a follow-up session at the turn of each season, so you'll have the information, tips and techniques to master the seasonal eating step of your wellness journey.

My clients know the power of foods in maintaining health and wellness. Checking in on the best power foods for you at the best times of the year ensures that you maintain that power edge indefinitely. Be proactive. Prevent rapid aging and disease later in life. And enjoy greater wellness now. Four times a year, making this change is your gift to your self.

You can count on this. Every time you come in, you will walk away with something new and valuable for your success at this season and on THIS step of your wellness journey. Nutrition is always developing, cutting-edge research emerges, and I am constantly reading, researching and attending lectures and seminars to ensure I am providing you with the most up-to-date information out there.

Here are a few critical benefits to follow-up sessions:

- Keep you motivated and on track
- Create variety so you don't become bored with the foods you are eating
- Re-introduce foods that were initially eliminated to ensure you are maintaining balance
- Track your progress and see how your symptoms improve
- Determine if you overcame certain nutritional conditions such as hypoglycemia, food sensitivities and candidiasis

- Ensure you are transitioning your diets with the seasons so you maintain balance and prevent cravings and maintain wellness throughout the year
- Determine your metabolic type so you know exactly what ratio of proteins, fats and carbohydrates your metabolic body needs to fuel optimally
- Understand how Ayurvedic principles on nutrition can help keep your body in balance and know which foods to avoid to prevent imbalance
- Offer you support when you are feeling challenged by maintaining your nutritional lifestyle and provide understanding and awareness as to why you may be diverting
- Look at mind/body connection to food and overcome certain emotional attachments you may have with food
- Learn how to eat soulfully so you create a conscious connection to the power of foods
- Use food as medicine to adjust hormones, boost neurotransmitters, reduce inflammation and support detoxification once you receive your laboratory results from Dr. Hoffman

Sound Nutrition is a remarkable paradigm and you can be a part of it. Maximize what is available to you. I am only as available to you as you make me; your nutrition goes only as far as you take it; and your health is what you make it. Schedule your nutrition sessions as diligently as seeing your doctor, dentist, massage therapist, veterinarian for your pet, accountant, renewing your gym membership, or getting your automobile oil changed. Quarterly visits benefit you the most, so make them part of your yearly regimen. You'll be grateful you did. Most importantly, having seasonal follow-ups moves you away from a "diet mentality" and towards creating a nutritional lifestyle for eternity.

Most of my nutrition tips and nutritional consults are focused around the "what" of foods—what foods to eat and what foods to avoid for optimum wellness in the body. Eating healthy food is only half of the story of sound nutrition, though. Being in the ideal state to digest and assimilate food is the other half. Marc David points this out in one of the most inspiring articles I have read, "Eating From the Tree: Nutrition Lessons for the Scientific Soul,"

> ...We've removed nourishment from nutrition. In our valiant efforts to create a science of eating, we've lost a bit of soul... we've lost something that though invisible, is never the less essential for cellular health and replenishment.[1]

In our fast-paced, quick fix, microwave society we may know logically what to eat, but we certainly have forgotten how to eat. So sit back and relax, take some deep breaths and add value to your life by increasing your intake of five of the most enjoyable, essential nutrients that bring nourishment and vitality to both body and soul: Vitamins R, O, Q, T and A.

vitamin r—relaxation

The autonomic nervous system (ANS) is the master regulator of every metabolic pathway in the body. Good digestion depends on the ANS. When our bodies are not relaxed—when they are in a state of stress—one branch of the ANS (the sympathetic system), turns on and steps up activity to prepare the body for fight or flight. In this reactive state, the digestive system shuts down. Conversely, when our bodies are relaxed, the other branch of the ANS (the parasympathetic system) dominates and maximum digestive function occurs. As David notes:

The same part of the brain that turns on stress turns off digestion, and the same part of the brain that turns on the relaxation
response turns on full, healthy digestive power.[2]

This means that getting maximum nourishment from the foods
we eat depends on eating in a state of parasympathetic dominance. So, if maximum nourishment depends on digestive system
efficiency, and digestive system efficiency depends on parasympathetic system dominance, and parasympathetic system dominance depends on being relaxed when we eat, then relaxed eating
is a major gift to our own physical and soul wellness.

There is little doubt that a major contributing factor to North
Americans being the most malnourished people in the world is the
fact that we do not take the time to relax while we eat. Constant
over-work, over-stress and over-rush result in bodies characterized
by sympathetic reactivity. So we do not digest, assimilate and efficiently use the very nutrients we need for optimum wellness.

In Europe, on the other hand, it is culturally acceptable to take
leisurely lunches, leave business at the office and welcome company (rather than the business deal) to the tables. People take
time, sit, enjoy, embrace, relax and breathe—the essence of maintaining a parasympathetic state—and optimum nutritional value
from power foods. Perhaps this is why Europeans rank higher
in health and have lower rates of disease than North Americans.
Perhaps this is why increasing Vitamin R for Relaxation promises
greater wellness and quality of life.

vitamin o—oxygen

Wellness begins at the cellular level. For optimum cellular metabolism we breathe and oxygenate our blood cells. If that sounds
simple, it is. Breathing before and after eating not only oxygenates,

it relaxes; both of these effects of breathing enable that parasympathetic system to efficiently digest the food you eat and the nutritional value you receive from it. So take 10 deep belly breathes before and after eating. It will improve dramatically both metabolism and digestion. There's more! When you take one simple breath between each bite of food, you give the parasympathetic system another boost in efficiency.

Those who smoke tend to enjoy a cigarette after a meal. They often say it is because the cigarette relaxes them and helps keep the bowels moving. I invite you to consider whether it's actually the cigarette that provides the benefit. I suggest to you that it is the simple task of sitting back, resting for a few minutes and taking deep breaths after a meal that triggers the relaxation response and peristalsis flow of the bowels.

vitamin t—time

One of the most common excuses for poor nutrition that I hear is, "I don't have time to eat." My response to that is, "you don't have time because you don't make the time." When you look at what and how you eat, and then link nutrition to your own highest values (reread Tip 18), you come to know with certainty that there simply is no other option but to take time to eat. Your nutrition is the foundation and essence of who you are, and provides you the vehicle to achieve what you desire in your life. If you do not take the time to build your foundation, then you are merely eating a diet with little nutritional value and void of nourishment. Time is a key component to your mastery of both nutrition and nourishment. Remember always to build your day around your nutrition as opposed to squeezing your nutrition into your day. Time for eating and breathing and relaxing nourishes a life—Vitamins T and O and R….

vitamin q—quality

I always advise you to eat a whole-foods clean diet. That is because your foods determine the essence of who you are. We resonate with the same frequency and energy that we ingest. In other words, the quality and magnetic energy of our food determines the vibrancy, energy, color (aura) and life spark that we emit. Foods that grow and subsist in nature are live, quality foods. Fast food, microwave food, processed, manufactured and packaged foods are dead foods. They have no quality, energy, color or vibrancy. Often they are loaded with toxicity, which further diminishes the nourishment of our cells. Those who eat such foods resonate with that same grey dead energy. Vitamin Q plays a significant role in our nourishment since the quality of our food dictates the health of our cellular body. So don't settle for less than quality foods.

vitamin a—awareness

Awareness, the state of being present…This is where our senses come to play. Simply tasting, smelling, visualizing and being present with our meals is one of the most significant steps we can take to ensure we are digesting, metabolizing, absorbing and getting full benefit and nourishment from what we are eating. David notes the significance of awareness to health in his article as he writes:

> As much as 30–40% of the total digestive response to any meal is due to the Cephalic Phase Digestive Response—our full awareness of what we're eating.[3]

If we are not aware, not only do we digest at 60–70% efficacy, we do not experience the feeling of being satisfied. If the brain does not experience the senses, it will not register satisfied or satiated, and overeating may result. Most people who say they have an overeating problem don't. According to David,

Their problem is that they fail to eat when they eat. They simply are not present with their meals and fail to satisfy the Cephalic Phase Digestive Response requirement—full awareness of what they are eating. This is what results in a continued longing for food.[4]

Awareness includes being present to where we are eating just as much as what we are eating. What does this mean? Quite simply, eating in front of the TV or computer, or eating while working, driving or talking on the phone leaves no room for awareness or the state of being present to the simple pleasure and enjoyment of eating. In contrast, if we sit, relax and set a calm, peaceful environment for meals, we increase our ability to nourish both body and soul.

So my friends, I urge you to make these vitamins a part of your daily nutritional lifestyle.

- Vitamin R: RELAX and eat in a parasympathetic state.
- Vitamin O: OXYGENATE your cells and breathe before, during and after your meals.
- Vitamin T: Take TIME to eat and nourish.
- Vitamin Q: Choose high QUALITY foods that are as close to their natural state as possible.
- Vitamin A: Be AWARE, present and grateful for and during every meal.

David's article reminded me of the connection between body and soul, and inspired me to "doctor the soul of the eater." Taking these five essential nutrients keeps the love and soul in the act and experience of eating. Nutrition is the science; nourishment is the soul. Merging these two truths forges the key to helping you achieve optimum wellness.

No matter what you did or didn't eat during the holiday season, remember this: It is not so much what we eat from Christmas to New Year's that matters; it is what we eat from New Year's to Christmas that is most important.

Following are twelve helpful "Back on Track" tips to motivate you to bring your nutritional lifestyle to the forefront again right now:

- Discard any holiday leftovers, desserts, chocolate, alcohol and other tantalizing foods.
- Book a follow-up sessions to adjust your nutritional lifestyle, get you back on track and keep you motivated.
- Review and implement your personal Nutritional Assessment and Recommendations.
- Re-read your value list so you have the purpose to go back to eating wisely. Ask yourself, how will not getting back on track be a drawback to my highest values?
- Spend some time at farmer's markets and health food stores and connect with wholesome food again.
- Restock your refrigerator with nutrient and magnetic rich foods, especially vegetables.
- Prepare meals and snacks to avoid restaurant eating.
- Give your digestive system a break. Eat light for one week: homemade soups, steamed vegetables, chicken stir-fry with cruciferous vegetables (kale, cabbage, Brussels sprouts, broccoli, cauliflower, bok choy), wild salmon, fruit, hard-boiled eggs and so on.
- For this one week, avoid red meats, excess nuts and seeds, dairy and grains; these are all heating foods and more difficult to digest.

- Over the course of each day, drink 1 ½ litres of room-temperature alkalinized water with lemon or liquid chlorophyll to cleanse your liver.
- Drink ginger tea throughout the day to cleanse your liver and support digestion.
- Fight the sugar cravings! Your body will be going through a slight sugar withdrawal because you likely have eaten more than usual in the past few weeks. Within one to three days, the cravings should disappear—that is, if you don't give in and you follow the steps from your customized programs!

If you are really feeling horrible after the holiday season try this easy, inexpensive, antioxidant-rich, immunity boosting, digestive-supporting and cleansing soup:

holiday hang-over soup

1 small–medium head organic green cabbage, shredded
2 large organic tomatoes, diced
2 small organic yellow or sweet onions, diced
2 organic red delicious apples, peeled and diced
7 cloves of garlic, thinly sliced
2–3 tbsp ginger root, thinly sliced
3 bay leaves

1 Put all ingredients in large pot. Fill pot with alkalinized water, so water just covers the ingredients.
2 Bring to a boil and boil for 45 minutes, reduce heat and simmer for 30 minutes.
3 Allow soup to cool and refrigerate. Reheat over the stove (not the microwave) as needed and enjoy it throughout the week!

Dr. Nicholas Perricone, in his superb book, *The Perricone Promise,* describes a conversation he had with a woman he had met at one of his lectures. The story offers valuable insight into some fundamental nutritional truths.

The majority of people, especially women, eat with weight in mind—not complexion or health. Many people choose food based on calories, carbohydrate content and fat grams. When diet consciousness (ye olde diet mentality) reigned, knowing food "numbers" was considered far more important than food quality, or the health and vibrancy of food. If you recall in Tip 34, I wrote about the reality that diet consciousness is coming to a close and we are changing rapidly the way in which we eat and view our nutritional lifestyles. This was the exact truth Perricone expressed in his story.

The woman in the story ate rice cakes because they have no calories. That fact alone, she thought would make them a healthy snack and prevent any weight gain. Rice cakes, as Perricone points out, are far from innocent food. They are high on the glycemic index (GI) and so rapidly convert to sugar. When they are puffed (as in puffed rice cakes), they skyrocket off the glycemic index charts. In fact, the GI of puffed rice cakes is higher than that of table sugar! Eating foods that are low in calories, but high on the GI generates the insulin response that causes us to store fat rather than burn it. Most importantly, this triggers a pro-inflammatory response in the body, which over time can lead to wrinkled skin, weight gain and "silent" inflammation that will mask itself as chronic disease.

With the science of anti-aging on the rise, we now know that "silent" inflammation is one of the most significant underlying factors in the development of chronic disease and rapid aging. The promising news is that sound nutrition is one of the most important pillars we have to reverse "silent" inflammation (which is why the

nutritional programs I design for you in Step Two implement essential anti-inflammatory nutritional principles).

It is time for a change in the way in which we think about food
and eating! If we want to prevent disease and slow the aging process, then we must eat foods that embody the characteristics that
make food anti-inflammatory and that create health in the body as
opposed to trigger disease.

The point is this: In this new nutrition paradigm, we know that it
is food quality that counts!

So what are characteristics to look for when it comes to choosing food? Quality, vibrancy, magnetic energy, color energy, nutrient availability and natural life force.

Consider the puffed rice cake as a case in point. It is manufactured in a food factory, refined, processed, stripped of vital
nutrients, until finally it is grey in color and dead in energy. It is an
empty food. In other words, it provides no benefit to the health of
our bodies. In contrast, a snack of sliced bright orange peppers,
deep green English cucumber and garlic infused hummus offers
energy, quality, nutritive power and magnetism that bring life spark
and health to our cells.

There is a full spectrum of colorful antioxidant and nutritive rich
foods to choose from (fish, buffalo, nuts, seeds, legumes and of
course our antioxidant-rich fruits and vegetables). These foods are
gifts from nature, and if incorporated as part of our daily nutritional
lifestyles, they can play one of the most significant roles on our
journey to optimum wellness. Perricone suggests that we "shop
thinking that each trip will be a new adventure",[1] and that there is
power in grocery shopping with purpose.

I often hear people say there is not enough variety or they are
bored with what they are eating. I wonder, then, if they are eating
more grey foods than vibrant foods, because there is an abundance of food choices with infinite health benefits. As Perricone

offers, "you will enjoy great health and culinary benefits when you choose foods imbued with the myriad hues of the rainbow."[2]

I always teach you to tap into how foods make you feel. Get connected to the quality, vibrancy, magnetic energy, color energy, nutrient availability and natural life force of the foods you choose to eat. Eat foods based on energy content not numbers. Leave the diet consciousness or diet mentality in the dust and live the expanding nutritional paradigm of the globe. There is no limit to the array of health-promoting and delicious foods available. So reject the dead foods and embrace the live. Your greatest reward will be the quality of your health—and your life.

"One cannot think well, live well, sleep well, if one has not dined well." –Virginia Woolf

The winter season always seems so long, especially when the next cold weather blast hits. Motivation to go to the gym dives, the will to cook healthy meals falters, and the desire to hibernate soars. This is opportunity! Now is the time to create variety in your diet. Variety now is very important. It is what will motivate you to maintain your nutritional lifestyle throughout the season.

Here are a few recipes to help you switch it up, try some new foods and tastes and keep you loving the joy of eating well.

herbed lemony lamb chops

4 lamb shoulder chops
1 tsp gated lemon peel
½ tsp rosemary
1 tsp oregano
1 tsp tarragon
3 tbsp lemon juice
1 tbsp tamari soy sauce

1 Heat large skillet over medium heat. Brown lamb chops on both sides.
2 Combine herbs, lemon peel, lemon juice and tamari in small bowl. Cover and simmer over medium–low heat for 20–25 minutes, or until tender.

buffalo chili[1]

1 tbsp coconut oil
½ cup onions, chopped
2 med garlic cloves, chopped

1 ½ cups celery, chopped

1 cup green pepper, chopped

1 ½ lb ground buffalo

2 tsp thyme

2 tsp chili powder

2 tsp ground cumin

1 tsp sea salt

1 8-oz can organic tomatoes

1 12-oz jar prepared salsa (organic ideally)

1. In large pot on medium–high heat, add oil and sauté onions, garlic, celery and peppers until translucent, 3–4 minutes.
2. Add ground meat and spices to pot and cook 5–6 minutes, stirring occasionally.
3. Pour salt, tomatoes and salsa into pot. Cover, reduce heat and simmer for 1 hour.
4. Serve into bowls over tiny steamed cauliflowerettes.

speedy zucchini

4 medium zucchini, sliced

2 large garlic cloves, finely chopped

2 tbsp ghee, butter or coconut oil

½ tsp basil

Dash of pepper and sea salt

1. Heat oil or butter in large frying pan over medium–high heat.
2. Add garlic and basil and cook until garlic sizzles. Add the zucchini and stir. Turn down heat to medium–low and cook for about 3 minutes, or until they can be easily pierced with a fork.
3. Season with sea salt and pepper.

Enjoy and happy winter cooking!

In Calgary we are blessed with unbearable cold snaps paired perfectly with the beautiful chinooks that follow. This is the time to get outside for a 30–45 minute walk and let eyes and skin absorb that vitamin D from the sun. It helps keep away those winter blues, re-energizes the body and offers some crisp fresh air instead of heaters and dry indoor air. Make a daily walk your gift. Your body and well being will love you for it.

When we exercise and have a sound nutritional lifestyle, a happy synergy occurs between our physiology and biochemistry. The truth of the matter is we cannot reach optimum wellness if we ignore either half of that relationship.

If you have weight to lose or would like to maintain your ideal body weight, this synergy becomes even more important. In fact, experts now say that 60–90 minutes of exercise a day is required for people who are overweight.

Dr. Joseph Mercola advocates 90 minutes of daily exercise for the person who has weight to lose. This is a lot of exercise time, and it is required only because overweight individuals have accumulated an exercise debt that must be repaid. Once a normal weight level is achieved then one can reduce levels to 45 minutes three to four times a week for weight maintenance.

These 90-minutes can be split up throughout the day (two 45-minute sessions or three 30-minute blasts of intensity). The key to exercising is to make sure you are using it effectively. Mercola explains that there are three important variables of exercise to keep in mind:

- Length of time
- Frequency
- Intensity

Gradually increase the amount of time you are exercising to one hour a day and then (if need be) to ninety minutes a day. For weight loss, the frequency is daily. This is a treatment dose until weight and insulin levels are normalized. Once normalized, three to four times a week becomes the frequency.

In terms of intensity, you should exercise hard enough so that it is difficult to carry on a conversation or read a magazine. However, if you cannot carry on a conversation AT ALL, then you have gone too far and need to decrease the intensity. Another way to determine if your intensity is too high is if you suddenly get a drop in body temperature or goose bumps.

Some of my clients have a long journey to take and often feel discouraged if weight doesn't melt off the way so many high-sales diet books suggest. Don't let feelings of discouragement weigh you down! I urge you to assess your workout regimens and ask yourself if there is more that you can do to create synergy between your physiology and your biochemistry. Are you meeting the latest recommendations? Are you doing the right exercise for your body type? Are you revving up a sluggish metabolism by exercising at high intensity every day? If you are a kapha body type, your weight loss will come much slower than a pitta or vata type, so this is particularly important for you.

Exercise is not just for weight loss. We know the extensive benefits of exercise include detoxifying the body. Our skin is the largest organ and one of the greatest eliminatory pathways for toxins. Exercise will definitely speed up necessary detoxification, since the more you sweat the more you excrete. This is especially important in our environmentally toxic world. Toxins cause us to hold on to body fat so the less you sweat and the more you hold on to toxins, the more difficult it will be to reach your ideal body weight.

Though we live in a society that looks for the quick fix, there is none when it comes to natural weight loss and the ability to achieve optimum wellness. There is no pill. Changing and evolving your nutritional lifestyle is not an easy task, but then great rewards come to those who act. The same holds true for exercise. Create the synergy!

for the love of meat!

"So, let's just describe the field of nutrition as it simply is: fresh, young, exciting, chaotic, uncertain and guaranteed to evolve and change. If you're looking for a unified voice from the community of experts as to the one true clinically and experienced validated perfect way for all humans to eat, expect to be disappointed."
–Marc David

With confusion surrounding saturated fats, growing fear of BSE and Avian flu and hormone and antibiotic injected cattle, more and more people are shunning meat and considering life as a vegetarian. But before you turn your back on your love for meat, consider the following nutritional truths.

It has now been widely accepted by scientists, doctors, nutritionists and other wellness practitioners that excess sugar and carbohydrate consumption is what leads to Syndrome X (obesity, insulin resistance, Type II diabetes, high cholesterol and high triglycerides) as a result of the overuse and overproduction of the hormone insulin. For years, saturated fat was considered the leading culprit for many of the chronic diseases in North America, but as Dr. Joseph Mercola writes in his *Total Health Cookbook and Program*, more and more research is showing us that in fact,

> Our body actually requires moderate levels of saturated fat to protect the arteries, process calcium, stimulate the immune system, and add structural stability to the cell and intestinal walls.[1]

In a lecture, Dr. Dean Rosedale, a leading healer in obesity, heart disease and diabetes, noted that we are responsible for creating a high saturated fat diet by feeding our animals too much grain. We North Americans ingest higher levels of saturated fat by eating second-generation carbohydrates from our animal protein. It is not the nature of cattle to have high levels of saturated fat; it is what we feed the animals to fatten them up for human consumption that increases saturated fat levels. This negatively affects our health. Biologically, the natural diet for cows is grass, not corn and grains. So, just as North Americans are overweight and have higher levels of cholesterol and triglycerides than ever before due to the over-consumption of grains and sugars, the same is true of our cattle in terms of obesity.

According to Rosedale, "There is a great deal of difference between a non-grain fed cow and a grain-fed cow. Non-grain fed will only have 10% or less saturated fat. Grain-fed can have over 50% saturated fat."[2] A non-grain fed cow and other grass-fed animal protein, such as game meat, will also have higher levels of omega-3 fatty acids and lower levels omega-6 fats (which can help to reduce "silent" inflammation). So for those who have been concerned about eating meat, know that consuming moderate amounts of the low saturated fat and high omega-3 ratios found in grass-fed animal protein, especially in game meat, is safe for those with inflammatory conditions or chronic diseases as well as for anyone interested in reaching optimum wellness.

Our patients and clients at the Hoffman Centre for Integrative Medicine who eat high quality, grass-fed and organic meat achieve excellent health results when they combine this food choice with other essential sound nutritional principles.

The fear and uncertainty surrounding the feeding and inject-ing of cows (with hormones and antibiotics) has driven more and more people to purchase organic and grass-fed animal protein and adventuring into the amazing taste and health benefits of wild game meat.

Meats such as buffalo, elk, ostrich and other game meat are nutritionally superior to skinless chicken breast, pork chops and lean beef. They are low in saturated fat (5%) and cholesterol and high in protein, iron, zinc, B12 and essential fatty acids. Moreover, according to the USDA handbook, one serving of bison (buffalo) meat provides 34% of the daily recommended amounts of protein, 32% of zinc, 33% of iron, 10% of niacin, 20% of phosphorus, 14% of vitamin B6 and 42% of selenium.

Game meats feed on grass alone and are not force-fed grains in feedlots. This makes game meat a non-allergenic, easy-to-digest food source for those with gluten or corn sensitivities or compromised digestion. Game meat is also free of all hormones and antibiotics typically found in the commercial meat you buy at your local grocery store.

Animal proteins are in fact good for you if you are eating the right kind. Quality (Vitamin Q) is the key to your healthy ingestion, digestion and assimilation of meat. It is important to find a source you trust when purchasing your meat, where staff is knowledgeable and take pride in offering you the best for your health. In Calgary Second to None Meats, Horizon Meats, farmer's markets and local health food stores are prime sources.

Following is a list of meats I recommend for all of my clients (depending on their body types):

- Free range and certified organic chicken
- Free range and certified organic turkey
- Free range and certified Cornish game hen
- Free range and certified organic eggs
- Certified organic and grass-fed beef
- Certified organic and grass-fed lamb
- Wild buffalo
- Wild elk
- Wild venison
- Wild ostrich

- Wild pheasant
- Wild quail
- Wild duck

Remember: Not all proteins have the same effect in every body. Know your Ayurvedic and metabolic type because some people need to base their intake around low-fat, light proteins (white poultry, light fish and dairy), while others thrive on high-fat, high purine proteins (dark poultry, beef and game meat). Determining your body type will take the guesswork out of meat selection so you can trust that what you are eating is what will create balance and optimum wellness in your body. Many people avoid eating meat because they believe it will cause acidity in the body. This is an over-generalization. Your metabolic type determines whether or not meat will create an acidic or alkaline environment in your unique body. For protein types meat is actually alkaline whereas it will create acidity for carbohydrate types.

There are safe and healthy alternatives to commercial meat that will support you as you journey to optimum wellness. You don't have to become a vegetarian. You can eat meat at ease knowing that you will not hinder your health by doing so. So all you health conscious meat lovers, think quality, lose the fear and bring back the love!

cooking with game meat

Now you know that quality meat is good for the body and soul, here are two recipes that use game meat that will help you put theory into practice.

beef, buffalo or venison stew with rosemary[3]

1 cup finely chopped onion
1 large garlic clove, minced

1 tbsp butter

2 ½ cups homemade or organic beef broth

1 lb lean stewing organic grass-fed beef, buffalo, or venison, cut into bite-sized pieces

1 15-oz can salt-free tomato sauce

2–4 large carrots, sliced

2 large celery stalks, sliced

2 cups green beans cut into 2-inch pieces

1 large rutabaga, diced, and/or 2–4 parsnips, sliced, and/or 1 lb potatoes, scrubbed and cut into 2-inch cubes

1 tsp dried rosemary leaves

½ tsp dried thyme leaves

1 large bay leaf

½ tsp sucanat (optional)

½ tsp Celtic Sea salt

½ tsp freshly ground black pepper

½ cup cold water

2 tsp arrowroot powder or kudzu

1   In a large heavy pot, melt the butter with 3 tablespoons of the broth, add the onion and garlic and cook, stirring, over medium heat, about 5 minutes or until onion is tender.

2   Add the meat and cook, stirring until the meat is just lightly browned on all sides.

3   Add the remaining broth and the tomato sauce. Stir to mix well. Add carrots, celery, green beans, rutabaga and parsnips. Stir in the rosemary, thyme, bay leaf, sucanat, salt and pepper. Bring to a boil. Cover, reduce heat and simmer 1 ½ hours, stirring occasionally. Remove bay leaf.

4   Stir arrowroot or kudzu in cold water. Bring stew to a boil. Add arrowroot or kudzu mixture, stirring until stew thickens slightly. Reduce heat and cook an additional 2 to 3 minutes.

ostrich stir-fry[4]

1 lb ostrich filets, cut into 1 ½-inch pieces
2 tbsp coconut oil
2 med garlic cloves
1-inch piece ginger, sliced
1 small leek, washed and cut into rings
4 cups shredded Chinese cabbage
8-oz button mushrooms, halved
1 med red pepper, cut into strips
1 10-oz pkg fresh snow peas diagonally cut in half
1 tbsp tamari soy sauce

1 Heat wok over medium high heat. Add coconut oil, ginger, garlic and leek and sauté until leek starts to wilt.
2 Add ostrich meat and sauté for 1–2 minutes. Remove meat from pan, place in bowl covered. Remove ginger slices.
3 Add Chinese cabbage and mushrooms to pan and stir-fry until cabbage starts to wilt. Add red peppers and snow peas. Stir-fry for 1–2 minutes more. Add ostrich.
4 Remove from heat and add tamari and stir to combine. Serve stir-fry immediately.

tealicious!

"Better to be deprived of food for three days, than tea for one."
–Chinese Proverb

From the rainforests of South America, to the veldt of South Africa and the green fields of Asia come some of the worlds most powerful and healthiest of all teas, which can be incorporated regularly into your nutritional lifestyle.

yerba maté

This South American tea is extremely high in antioxidants that promote health by neutralizing harmful chemicals in the body. Antioxidants in Maté have been shown to reduce the risk of cancer and heart disease, as well as slow the aging process.

Yerba Maté also has high levels of chromium in it, which may be why this tea is known to be an appetite suppressant. It increases metabolism and is thermogenic. "Thermogenic" means that it actually induces the body to burn calories making Maté a great supporter for weight loss. This is a rare quality that most other types of tea do not possess.

antioxidant power*

Yerba Maté	5102
Black tea	2947
Green tea	2701

* Expressed as the ORAC value, which measures the ability of an antioxidant to scavenge harmful free radicals.

green tea

From Asia comes green tea, which has many significant medicinal as well as therapeutic health benefits. It is anti-inflammatory, lowers blood cholesterol levels, has a beneficial effect on circulation and the liver, protects against tooth decay, increases mental clarity, protects the brain from Alzheimer's disease and detoxifies the blood. The polyphenols and high antioxidant content in green tea may inhibit the growth of cancer cells and the development of tumors. Green tea does contain caffeine so if you are sensitive pour a little water over the leaves prior to infusion and strain the water off after 30 seconds. Then prepare the tea as usual.

white tea

White tea, also from Asia, comes from green tea but it goes through very little processing (steaming, rolling, oxidation) which keeps the cell structure of the tea leaves virtually unaltered. This purity is what is believed to cause white tea to have a greater concentration of antioxidants than all of the teas that originate from green tea. White tea also only has 5 mg of caffeine per cup compared to 20 mg in green tea and 50 mg in black tea.

rooibos tea

This South African tea contains 50% more antioxidants than green tea making it a wonderful choice for an anti-inflammatory and cancer fighting diet. Rooibos tea also has antispasmodic properties that can help ease colic and stomach cramps. It is also beneficial in aiding in the relief of skin problems such as eczema, skin rashes and acne. Rooibos tea is also a rich source of minerals as it contains calcium, potassium, zinc, iron, sodium, fluoride, magnesium and manganese.

african fruit iced tea[1]

8 rooibos tea bags
4 stalks organic mint
1 organic lemon
1 organic orange

2 slices organic ginger

1 tbsp honey (optional)

1   Fill a 1-litre container or jug (with a seal) with cold spring water. Add tea bags and set aside.
2   Slice lemon and orange into ½-inch round slices. Keep the rind intact.
3   Peel and grate ginger in large shaved pieces.
4   Add lemon, orange, ginger and mint stalks to tea. Refrigerate for 30–45 minutes.

Drink to your health!

It's that time again. On the brink of a new season we need to transition our diets. Seasonal eating is one of the most important pieces to your nutritional mastery and in helping you stay balanced throughout the year.

Every season, Mother Nature provides us with the very foods we need to keep the body balanced and supported. For example in the cold winter months, we are gifted with root vegetables that are heavy and heating to keep us insulated throughout the cold season. In the spring these vegetables fade and the sprouts and bitter greens arrive to help us clear excess mucous and toxicity we accumulated in the winter. They also support liver detoxification, blood purification and fat burning metabolism that is imperative to take place at this time of year. In summer, we receive sweet and cool foods to counter the heating qualities of the season.

There is purpose to the foods that are available at every season. If you fail to compensate for changes in the seasons and if you are not even connected to seasonal foods then you have the potential to set your body up for great imbalance, disease and disharmony. The junctions between seasons are common times to fall ill, so be preventative and make the transition.

There are specific vegetables and herbs you need to incorporate into your diet at different times of year. Certain fruits are more beneficial than others. In some seasons the need for grains is less and the consumption of legumes increases. Some proteins are better than others and the amounts and types of fats you consume also vary from season to season. Even your daily exercise and lifestyle need to be adjusted at each quarterly transition.

Spring is the time of year to ensure you are resetting your fat metabolism, detoxifying your liver and gallbladder with specific cleanses and revitalizing the body, mind and spirit. It is the season that sets the body up properly for the rest of the year. If you miss out on this opportunity then it is likely you will gain weight, struggle with weight loss throughout the year, create a sluggish and fatigued body, overburden your liver, weaken your immune system, catch more colds and flu, and dim your spirit.

You can't ignore the perfection and power of Mother Nature. To all of you who believe in the power of food and value your health, here is to balance throughout the year and embracing and enjoying your ultimate seasonal diet!

Many of you ask me how long it will take before you feel better, get results or reach your weight loss goals. That is often a difficult question to answer. Every body is different and has a unique blue-print. So what you can do to get an idea of the length of time it will take to make some change is to look into basic biochemistry.

What we do know: Blood cells have a 120-day lifespan. It takes four months for the cells to live, die and rebirth into stronger healthier cells or weaker diseased cells. It is this cellular turnover that you are looking for to make a significant change in the state of your overall health. Since the cells have 120 day life/death cycle, it would be wise to look ahead and set your first set of goals for the first four month cycle from the day you start your program (this includes an exercise program as well). If you have been on your program for a while, then mark the four-month cycles by the first day of every season.

The first four-month cycle is about cleaning up the body, putting in new fuel and getting the body used to new nutritional habits. So at the end of the first four months, your cellular body should be rebirthing into stronger healthier cells. But it is in the second four-month cycle when the cells finally have sufficient energy from new nutritional fuel to detoxify the body, support organ systems, burn body fat more efficiently and create more alkalinity in the body. Imagine how your cellular health will make you feel in the third four-month cycle: higher energy, clearer and brighter eyes, sharper mental activity, stronger physical body and balanced emotional health. By the end of the fourth four-month cycle, you will have hit a one-year cellular turnover. This is the point of true rejuvenation, vibrancy and radiance.

For optimum wellness to be achieved a full year cellular turn-around needs to take place within the body. That may sound like a long time (especially in a microwave society where we want a quick fix for everything and anything). When it comes to your health, however, you can't fight the biochemistry. It is what it is and all you can do is support and surrender to the wisdom of the 120-day cycles.

In this case, what you don't know can indeed hurt you. Become aware of and remember when your four-month cycles end because this seems to be the time when people fall off programs, stop going to the gym and revert back to old habits. I am not sure why this happens. Perhaps a biochemical shift takes place within the body, but whatever the reason every four months an internal struggle occurs between staying the course and giving up. This may well be true for everything in life—we may get tired at work, hit an emotional low, leave a project that we have been working on, gravitate towards different people socially, end relationships and feel anxious or antsy without apparent cause.

There are two things you can do to transition into your next 120-day cycle successfully and avoid the "go on or give up" struggle.

1   Mark every four-month cycle in your calendar. Take a highlighter and make it very visible so when that four-month date approaches you remain conscious that a shift will take place. This is when you also determine to what extent you have met your last four-month goals and set up new goals for the next cycle. Notice if you are feeling better, stronger, healthier and more vibrant than in your last cycle. This awareness will give you the motivation to go another round. Just being conscious and aware of the 120-day cycle can be all it takes to prevent the drop-off.

2 This is where seasonal eating becomes significant. Interestingly enough, the seasons too go through three-four month cycles. Mother Nature and biochemistry seem to be working together on this one! It is one of the most important reasons why I teach you how to transition your diets seasonally and why seasonal eating is an integral part of my 7 Steps to Sound Nutrition™ program. If you connect with Mother Nature's cycles and change your diet and routine as the seasons change, it becomes much easier to stay committed to your newfound lifestyle. You enjoy variety with foods, look forward to eating foods you haven't seen since the previous year, notice that your body stays balanced while people around you (who are not as connected as you are) seem to be dropping off and getting sick. Being connected to the seasons is powerful. It's also a great motivator. In fact, you will feel that it is just natural to continue to move your body throughout each seasonal or cyclical change.

So now you know how long it will take to notice a difference in how you feel and in reaching your health goals. Commit to four, four-month cycles and seasonal transitions. During that time, choose to trust that your body is journeying to optimum wellness. After that first year your body will have fully embraced this new lifestyle and when you transition into year two and begin the seasons again, your body will know what to do naturally, and your cellular body will continue to birth stronger, healthier and more vibrant cells.

On the brink of the arrival of spring, the sun is shining, the birds are chirping and the air is crisp and fresh. As nature prepares for the turn of seasons so too, do our bodies.

We naturally feel the urge to be outside. We are antsy and waiting for that perfect moment to go for the first outdoor run of the season. We are spring cleaning our homes. We are coming out of hibernation and generally feel more social and outward. Certainly, we have noticed that the time has come to shed those five pounds of insulating winter weight.

It is during this transition that taste buds are changing and the body's innate wisdom is asking for more fruit, leafy green and bitter vegetables, and fresh organic vegetable juicing to cleanse the liver. We crave salads over soups and lighter, lower fat proteins over heavier purine proteins. We move away from root vegetables and gravitate towards sprouts, bitter greens and legumes. The body knows it is time to detoxify and build itself up again after the long winter season.

The body journeys through two six-month cycles. From September to February, the body actually destroys itself. We exercise less, exert less energy, stay indoors, reflect inwards, tend to more feelings of depression, develop dry skin and eat more sugar, along with heavier and comforting foods. But then from March to August, the body rebuilds itself. We are more active we absorb more vitamin D, feel lighter, outward, and happier; have more color in our faces, eat more fresh foods, eat lighter foods and naturally consume less sugar. This build and destroy cycle is the body's way of maintaining balance.

Like everything else in life, the body must go through its natural life/death/life cycle. Don't be hard on yourself if you feel like the winter months put you in a downswing. Trust that the upswing will always follow. The key is to stay in tune with these natural rhythms and support the body through both phases.

Think about your last six months and see where your body was mentally, physically, emotionally and spiritually. Look at the natural destroying rhythms your body went through. Perhaps you exercised less, ate more sugar, detoxified your body, eliminated unhealthy cells and toxins, removed amalgams, released emotional baggage, ended relationships, got less sunshine, and so on. Then, think about the next six months to come. Get excited about the rebuilding cycle your body is eager to go through. Set new goals for yourself. Ask yourself, "What do I want my body, mind and spirit to look like by the end of this six month life cycle?" This is the time for renewal and new beginnings.

Spring is about rebirth, rejuvenation and revitalization. As Dr. Elson Haas writes in *Staying Healthy With the Seasons,* "spring is the time for clearing the past, healing the present and planning for the future."[1] Know that your body is days away from beginning its natural rebuilding cycle. It is an exciting time, an uplifting time and a time for you to meet your health goals. This is also a great time to come in for a follow-up to adjust your individual nutritional needs so your body is supported and ready to birth its vitality yet again.

words of wisdom from the byrds

To everything (turn, turn, turn)
There is a season (turn, turn, turn)
And a time for every purpose, under heaven

A time to be born, a time to die
A time to plant, a time to reap
A time to kill, a time to heal
A time to laugh, a time to weep

To everything (turn, turn, turn)
There is a season (turn, turn, turn)
And a time for every purpose, under heaven

A time to build up, a time to break down
A time to dance, a time to mourn
A time to cast away stones, a time to gather stones together

To everything (turn, turn, turn)
There is a season (turn, turn, turn)
And a time for every purpose, under heaven

A time of love, a time of hate
A time of war, a time of peace
A time you may embrace, a time to refrain from embracing

To everything (turn, turn, turn)
There is a season (turn, turn, turn)
And a time for every purpose, under heaven

A time to gain, a time to lose
A time to rend, a time to sew
A time to love, a time to hate
A time for peace, I swear it's not too late

Juicing is a fantastic way to get live, pre-digested, magnetic-rich energy and nutrients into our bodies. Our need for vegetables is so high and many of us don't quite reach our daily requirements (ideally 4 cups a day), so juicing becomes an efficient way to pack a lot of goodness into one glass.

Spring is the best time to introduce juicing to your nutritional lifestyle. It is the season to focus on supporting and detoxifying the liver, to clear out excess mucus accumulated in the winter and to revitalize energy and cells for the six month building cycle (see Tip 44). One of the best ways to achieve all of this is by increasing the greens in your diet, especially the bitter leafy greens that naturally sprout and grow in the spring season. These vegetables contain high amounts of chlorophyll, vitamins K, A, E, B-vitamins, iron, potassium, sodium and magnesium, which are vital nutrients for the liver and cells. By juicing these magnetic and nutrient rich vegetables daily, you will do wonders for your liver and overall health.

You will find that as you juice, you will feel lighter, more vibrant, more energetic, and you'll even have a spring in your step! Juicing can be your greatest medicine after the long winter season when we are used to feeling heavy, weighed down, lazy and fighting the winter blahs.

important tips to consider when juicing

- Juice only organic produce. Never juice produce that has been sprayed with chemicals, pesticides or herbicides. The purpose of juicing is to detoxify and cleanse the liver; so juicing chemicals would only counteract that goal.
- Juice only vegetables that won't spike blood sugars. If you have higher glycemic vegetables (carrot, beet), ensure they make up the smallest amount of your juice and balance them

with leafy greens. If you combine fruits with your vegetable juice the best fruits to juice are lemons and limes. The rinds of these fruits also have potent antioxidants.

- If you have diabetes, insulin resistance, hypoglycemia, or obesity, juice only three–four times a week with green vegetables and ensure you eat some protein with your juice to slow the rate in which the natural sugars will enter your bloodstream.
- To prevent spikes in blood sugars and to maximize nutrient absorption (many nutrients in vegetables are fat soluble), have an essential fat such as a teaspoon of nut butter, ghee or your fish oil along with or in your juice.
- Juice only vegetables that support your metabolic type as not all vegetables are created equal or equally affect every body. If you have not yet determined your metabolic type, I highly recommend you come in for a session (or read *The Metabolic Typing Diet* by William Wolcott.)
- Juice daily as part of your nutritional lifestyle for the entire spring season.
- Juicing does not replace regular vegetable consumption— the fibre is not present in juicing. It is still important to get roughage from salads or steamed or stir-fried vegetables at lunch and dinner.
- Do not discard the fibre from the juicer—use it for soups or feed it to your pets.
- Juice in the morning upon waking, prior to showering and breakfast, or juice for a mid-morning and mid-afternoon snack. Do not replace a meal with juice.
- You can buy a juicer at Costco, Superstore and at some health food stores.

The following are some juicing recommendations for the spring.
You need a handful of each vegetable, unless otherwise noted.

- Parsley, broccoli and spinach
- Broccoli, cabbage and kale
- Chunk of ginger root, parsley, 1 clove garlic, ½ lemon and 1 carrot
- Fennel, spinach, celery and lime
- Beet tops, parsley, spinach, 1 carrot, ½ apple
- Parsley, 1 clove garlic, 1 carrot and celery
- Cucumber, beet, parsley, ½ lemon and spinach
- Wheatgrass and mint sprig
- Swiss chard, parsley, spinach, celery
- Cabbage, bok choy and celery
- Spinach, kale, beet greens, ½ lime and broccoli
- ½ beet, ½ apple, dandelion greens and kale

Mother Nature provides us with the right foods to support the health of our bodies at every season. I urge you to enjoy that magnificence and get connected to the natural rhythms and cycles that we are apart of. Juice this spring season and experience the incredible health benefits you will receive. It's all about the power of foods my friends!

ayurveda: the science of life

"The guiding principle of Ayurveda is that the mind exerts the deepest influence on the body, and freedom from sickness depends upon contacting our own awareness, bringing it back into balance, and then extending that balance to the body. This state of balanced awareness, more than any kind of physical immunity, creates a higher state of health." –Deepak Chopra

Dating back 5000 years, Ayurveda is an ancient form of healing and the oldest healing system. Ayurveda translates to "the science of life." It is a system that teaches how to achieve balance through diet, herbs, exercise and lifestyle choices based on your unique body type or dosha. According to this science, when imbalance exists in the body, mind and spirit disharmony results and "disease" develops. The purpose of Ayurveda is to eliminate blockages that create the disharmony so balance and wellness can be achieved. According to Ayurveda, the body consists of five different elements: earth, water, fire, air and space. These elements define who you are, how you act and why your body is the way and shape it is.

Ayurveda distinguishes three body types, called doshas. The dosha types are called vata, pitta and kapha.

Vata types are made up of the elements air and space. They are often tall, lean and "airy and spacey!" They are the movers and shakers, the ones who can do endless amounts in a day, and go all day and forget to eat; yet they are the ones who need to eat the most and have the most routine and structure to their day. If not grounded and balanced, vata types manifest with fatigue. They often have dry skin, are cold all the time and can be mentally and emotionally scattered. To bring the vata type back to balance we need to ensure that their nutritional lifestyles are full of essential fats and higher purine proteins to warm, lubricate and insulate their cold and dry elements. They would benefit from lots of chili, soups, stews and crock-pot meals and would want to avoid cold and dry foods (they are already too cold and dry). They would also benefit from meditation, Bikram yoga and saunas to ground and warm their body types.

Pitta types are made up of the elements fire and water. Pitta types are often a medium build with freckles and red or brown hair. They are often the leaders; they have direction and strong will. Often they are Type A personalities. They are always structured (and get impatient with scattered vata types!) and they are fiery! When pitta types get too stressed, overwhelmed, irritated or over-heated they create too much fire in their bodies and often manifest with inflammatory conditions. They often come in with red skin, heart conditions, arthritis, gout and overall "silent" inflammation in the body. To bring a pitta type back into balance we need to ensure that their nutritional lifestyles nourish with cool and bitter foods to pacify the fire within. We need to eliminate any foods that stoke the fire—such as excess red meat, pungent (hot, spicy) foods and alcohol. Swimming as a form of exercise may be a valuable part of a pitta lifestyle because the cool water would refresh and prevent or pacify the fire.

Kapha types are made up of the elements water and earth. They tend toward a heavier build, rounder face and a gentle predisposi-tion. They are the nurturers, care givers and often are stay-at-home mothers, teachers or nurses. They often are slow to start in the morning, have sluggish metabolism and find it very difficult to lose weight. Kapha types need constant variety, stimulation and regular vigorous cardiovascular exercise or they will put their bodies out of balance. Kapha types, if out of balance will often present with con-ditions of excess moisture such as candidiasis, edema, fluid reten-tion, high blood pressure and obesity. To come back into balance, kaphas need stimulating spices to get the metabolism moving, dry foods and only small amounts of oily moist food. Salads, vegetable juicing, chicken breasts with hot spices and high impact aerobics comprise an ideal lifestyle for a balanced kapha type.

Ayurveda is a fascinating tool that I work with in my practice. When I first meet with you in Step One of the 7 Step program, just by looking at you and listening to you speak, I have already assessed a great deal about who you are, why you manifested with the symptoms or conditions you have and how I can support you and what I can recommend in your nutritional lifestyle to pacify imbalances in your body. I assure you I'm not psychic; I just understand the science of life!

The purpose of Step Four of the 7 Step program, is for you to understand this science as well. When you understand your Ayurvedic dosha and the elements that make you up then you know how to create a lifestyle that will keep your elements in balance. You will know the foods most balancing for you and the foods that cause imbalances. You will have an understanding of how lifestyle choices can irritate or pacify your body type. You will learn which form of exercise and yoga would be best for you, always with the intention of keeping the body in balance. Even certain oils, herbs, scents and spices would be designated to your specific dosha to create harmony in body, mind and spirit.

There is true wisdom in this ancient form of healing. It has been said "knowledge becomes wisdom when it becomes your personal experience." By living true to the Ayurvedic principles you will begin to have a knowing about who you are and gain experience in what keeps you balanced and free of disease. That is wise living!

"You don't have to cook fancy or complicated masterpieces—just good food from fresh ingredients." –Julia Child

The following recipes will get you moving into spring. Enjoy all the foods you have not eaten since last spring, savor new tastes, try time-tested spices and herbs, and know that your food choices have the potential to support what nature intended this season— renewal, rejuvenation, rebirth, detoxification, lightness and spring in every step! Enjoy!

spring salad

This recipe is a nice way to reintroduce salads in the spring. Focus on bitter greens, sprouts, pumpkin seeds and turmeric— all-important foods for the season.

1 cup organic arugula or spring mix
8 organic pea pods
½ cup organic alfalfa or broccoli sprouts
12 organic black olives
1 organic artichoke heart
½ cup organic celery
1–2 tbsp organic pumpkin seeds
1 tsp turmeric
Drizzle of olive oil

1 In a nice salad bowl, mix the above ingredients.
2 Top salad with protein of choice (chicken breast, oven roasted turkey, chickpeas or wild salmon).

blended broccoli soup[1]

This is a great soup for a rainy spring day—warm, yet promoting those essential bitter greens for spring detoxification.

1 tbsp coconut oil
2 med green onions, coarsely chopped
2 cloves garlic, minced
1 tbsp basil leaves, dried
1 large head fresh broccoli, washed and chopped
2 cups chopped spinach, kale, collards, Swiss chard or other dark leafy greens
4 cups vegetable or chicken broth
2 cups coconut milk
1 tsp sea salt or kelp (seaweed)

1 In a large soup pot, sauté garlic and green onions in oil for 1–2 minutes. Add broccoli and stir.
2 Cook over medium heat, stirring until broccoli turns bright green. Add basil and additional chopped greens.
3 Cover and steam for 3–4 minutes.
4 Transfer vegetables into a food processor or blender (may need to do two batches). Add a little liquid and process until vegetables start to be smooth. Add remaining liquids and salt or kelp. Process until smooth.
5 Reheat gently if necessary. Serve with a protein of choice.

cornell bbq sauce[2]

Fire up those barbecues with an easy and tasty nightshade and sugar free BBQ sauce.

1 cup coconut oil
2 cups cider vinegar

3 tbsp sea salt

2 tbsp poultry seasoning

½ tsp pepper

1 egg

1   In a heavy saucepan, combine oil, vinegar, poultry seasoning, salt and pepper. Bring to a boil, reduce heat and then simmer for 3–4 minutes.

2   Remove from heat. For a thicker sauce, quickly whisk in a beaten egg.

3   Let cool.

4   Store sauce in a glass jar with lid in refrigerator, if not using right away. Keeps up to 2 months. Use this as a marinade for chicken or turkey.

ideal spring dinners

- Broiled trout rubbed with ginger, cinnamon, anise, turmeric.
- Sautéed mixed greens (dandelions, spinach, mustard greens) with garlic and a drizzle of olive oil.
- Wild rice cooked with turmeric, black pepper and ginger.
- Chicken, steamed broccoli with ghee and stir-fried Swiss chard and kale with garlic and ginger.
- Tilapia, lightly steamed fiddleheads with touch of ghee and lightly steamed carrots with coriander.
- Lamb, lightly steamed Brussels sprouts with touch of ghee and stir-fried dandelion greens in garlic with turmeric.

creative spring salads

- Spring mix or arugula, parsley, celery, sprouts, olives and lentils with tahini.
- Purple cabbage, shredded carrot, parsley, raisins and chick peas with lemon juice and hemp oil.

- Arugula, spring mix or dandelion greens, pumpkin seeds, dried cranberries, artichoke hearts, chicken breast with flax oil and turmeric.
- Spinach, asparagus tips, pomegranate seeds, green onion, sunflower seeds, tilapia with olive oil, dill and lemon juice.

Happy spring eating!

Do you ever feel discouraged that you are not achieving the weight loss or health goals that you set out for yourself? Are you caught up by the numbers the scales dictate to you every day? Do you stress over taking your supplements at the exact right time and right dose? Do you worry about when you are going to get to the grocery store to buy the foods you need to fuel on throughout the week? Have you created more stress around implementing a sound nutritional lifestyle and creating a health regimen, than you have embraced and enjoyed the experience of it? Have you lost sight of why you set out on your journey to optimum wellness in the first place?

To all of you who may feel discouraged or frustrated because you have not yet reached your goals, I urge you to surrender. Now, before you put that coffee and muffin in your mouth, I don't mean to give up! I mean surrender to the experience. Consider that you put more pressure on yourself by thinking about what you have not accomplished yet, and not acknowledging all that you have.

On your journey to optimum wellness it is so important that you focus on being present. Acknowledge the successes you have achieved. Don't feel discouraged by the long road ahead or challenges you may feel you still have to tackle.

Perhaps if we surrender to the experience and just appreciate the journey, we will ease up on ourselves and find that we are indeed achieving results. Our results may even come faster when we are not putting so much pressure on ourselves. After all, they do say, the water doesn't boil any faster by staring at it!

I wonder if the stress we create by stepping on the scale, being meticulous about every detail of our program, and focusing on what we want our bodies to have and look like, prevents us from celebrating what we have accomplished to date and accepting what is, as it is, today. Perhaps we need to trust the innate intelligence of our body, that it will get to where it needs to go in its due course and not when we mandate it to.

Just focus on surrendering. Stop trying to control the process and just let the process happen. Acknowledge where you were before you started your new nutritional lifestyle and then be grateful for where you are now. Know that achieving optimum wellness is not finite. Optimum wellness is an infinite journey and a lifelong commitment of ups and downs, challenges and successes, health and disease. So ease up, and just let it happen and trust that your body and experience will all unfold as it should. Surrender, surrender, surrender...

Lovin' its contribution to life.... Olive oil protects against cardio-vascular disease, lowers high cholesterol, decreases constipation and stomach upset, furthers liver detoxification by promoting bile secretion, reduces gallstones, helps membrane development and cell formation, reduces some cancers as well as rheumatoid arthritis, dry skin and stretch marks! Extra virgin olive oil is indeed one of the super oils. I recommend you include it regularly in your sound nutritional lifestyle.

Olive oil contains 77% monounsaturated fatty acids, 14% saturated fatty acids and 9% polyunsaturated fatty acids, plus vegetable mucilage, vitamin E and A, carotene, chlorophyll, magnesium, phytosterols, squalene (potent antioxidant that protects oil from going rancid) and many other nutritive components that promote good health.

One of the excellent truths about olive oil is that it does not upset the critical omega-3:6 ratio; most of the fatty acids in olive oil are actually omega-9. This is extremely important in your quest for optimum wellness as an imbalance of essential fatty acids triggers a host of chronic diseases, autoimmune diseases, and speeds up the aging process. So to ensure you have the right balance of omega-3:6:9 use other oils mentioned in Tip 53 along with your beneficial olive oil.

Monounsaturated fats such as olive oil are not as easily damaged by oxygen as other types of fat. The monounsaturated fats are more stable than polyunsaturated fats (vegetable oils). Because olive oil also contains the important antioxidant vitamin E, it is even more protected from oxidation and free radical damage. These facts hold true in the cold state and do not extend to cooking and heating at high temperatures.

According to Udo Erasmus in *Fats That Heal Fats That Kill,* when olive oil is heated above 150˚C, it loses its protective and nutritive effects. But Erasmus does conclude, "olive oil is acceptable for low-temperature frying/cooking."[1] In Dr. Joseph Mercola's opinion, "olive oil is a healthy fat to include in your diet in a non-heated form but it is not the best oil to cook with, as it is highly susceptible to oxidative damage when heated."[2] Some labels on olive oil now include a warning to cook with olive oil only on low heat and never on high heat. When cooking at high temperatures, it is better to use saturated fats (coconut, ghee and butter) or macadamia nut oil because they are less susceptible to oxidation and free radical damage.

Other important tips: only use olive oil that is labeled extra virgin and organic. Together, these labels assure you that the oil has been cold-pressed from freshly harvested olives and contains no harmful pesticides or chemicals. Ensure your olive oil is unrefined and unheated, which is what makes it a healthy oil compared to vegetable oils. Keep your olive oil in an opaque jar to minimize oxidation from light. In my opinion, the best place for olive oil is drizzled over a magnetic-rich, color-full, antioxidant-rich salad.

Try these applications for olive oil from the *Complete Guide to Natural Healing*:[3]

- To prevent hair loss—Massage scalp with olive oil every evening for eight days. Let it work overnight and wash it out in the morning.
- For constipation—In morning take one teaspoon of olive oil mixed with lemon juice on an empty stomach.
- To moisturize skin—Apply daily to dry spots or stretch marks.

You've got your bags packed, cosmetics loaded, passport and airline ticket in hand, your confirmation number for your hotel, contact numbers for while you are away, your briefcase and lap top for your business meeting and you're set. Or are you? The one thing you need the most, you are leaving behind—your fuel!! And by doing so, you are leaving your energy, production, health and vitality in the hands of other people. Now, why would you do that?

Traveling and eating well can often be difficult. But, if you plan ahead and put as much time, effort and thought into what you'll be eating while away as you do in planning your trip, you can actually travel the nutritionally sound way. The following are some tips to help you do just that!

Many international flights and longer distance North American destinations are now offering many meal options based on medical and religious needs (Air Canada has 17 options!). You can now order a diabetic meal (high protein meal), vegetarian or even a gluten or lactose free meal. So when booking your flights, ask about the meal choices you have and ask for an alternative to the typical high glycemic nutrient void foods you usually receive.

On shorter flights, bring your own food and bottled water with you. They often don't serve anything so bring your own snacks from home so you don't go hours without eating.

Bring your protein powder with you or a meal replacement drink from the health food store (measure out enough and keep it in a Ziploc baggie so you don't have to bring the whole canister). You can purchase mini portable hand blenders and make your shakes in your hotel room. If you feel that is too much effort, make friends with the bar tender (i.e. tip him/her well) and ask him/her to blend up your protein powder, with ice and water (go to the market or grocery store around the corner from where you are staying and pick up a banana to throw in as well).

Go to the grocery store while away. Little markets or health food stores often have salad bars, fresh made deli meats (oven roasted chicken or turkey), BBQ chickens, olive bars, nuts and seeds, yogurt, cottage cheese, pre-cut vegetables and fruit. Buy a bag of groceries and keep it in your room (store it in the mini-bar) to have for snacks or mini-meals. This is ideal if you want to avoid a continental breakfast pre-meeting and don't have enough time to go to a restaurant.

Now, I know the continental breakfast is free but without doubt, you will feel like hell when you're done—bagels, toast, cereal, muffins, danishes and artificially sweetened non-fat yogurt. White death! You'll be hypoglycemic within one hour. It is really not worth it. Go to the hotel restaurant or diner around the corner and pay for an egg and veggie omelet. For an extra $10.00 your body, mind and spirit will thank you for it, so don't cheap out on your health!

Pack a cooler (especially ideal if taking a road trip). Bring fresh fruit, cut up veggies and hummus, natural jerky, hard boiled eggs, trail mix, dried fruit, cans of wild salmon, albacore chunk light tuna (lowest source of mercury in tuna fish), sardines or yogurt.

Make your own homemade trail mix (raw unsalted almonds, sesame seeds, cashews, walnuts, shredded coconut, raisins) and bring it along with you. It makes for a great snack.

High quality protein bars are always ideal if going away. They are great to keep in your purse, brief case or hotel room. They are a great way to keep you satiated between meals or as another ideal alternative for the continental breakfast.

Ask the concierge of your hotel for some restaurant ideas. Explain the type of food you are looking for and you can be sure you will be sent in the right direction.

When ordering at a restaurant, assess the menu carefully. Always skip over the bread, sandwich, pasta and pizza options and look at the salads, soups and entrées. Always make substitutions and remember you are paying for the meal so you should receive a plate of food that you know will make you feel your best. Don't settle for their meal creation if you know it is not right for you. Create your own meal by mixing and matching foods on the menu so you can be certain you will feel good when leaving the restaurant. There is always something you will be able to eat.

If traveling in the U.S. only eat half of your plate. The serving sizes are ridiculous, so don't overeat like our fellow Americans! If in Asia, watch the white rice consumption. If not careful you can end up eating 4 cups a day, which is not good for the waistline. Only eat a third of what they give you, one meal a day.

Be aware of what is around you. Just like you would window-shop for clothes, window shop for food. There are many juice bars, soup shops, wraps, fresh food-to-go places popping up in every city. These are much safer options than any fast food restaurant.

Be adventurous! Many ethnic restaurants offer healthier meal choices than North American food. Go for Vietnamese, Japanese, Moroccan, Lebanese, Nepalese and Malaysian food. And vegetarian restaurants are often your healthiest choices with creative salads, homemade soups and bean dishes (most offer egg dishes so if you need animal protein, you should be covered).

If you do eat something you know is not the best for you, don't sweat it. Just tap in to how it makes you feel. Often times going away can offer us our greatest "aha" moments. You should be able to tell right away which foods trigger your symptoms. And if you dabble in the wrong foods enough times while away, you can be sure that once you get home you'll be dying to get back to your sound nutritional lifestyle!

So there you have it. It takes a little more effort but I'd say your health and well being is worth it. Why go away and feel awful? Your fuel is the most important thing you can have with you so do not forget to pack it!

"It is you who eats for you." –Unknown

Variety is the spice of life. It's also the key to preventing monotony with your nutritional lifestyle. The following list of meal ideas will energize you, keep you motivated, and ensure you are eating for the spring season, and remind you that eating well beats eating boring, dead food any day of the week.

Warning: Reading this list below may induce hunger pangs, gurgling stomachs and salivary excretions!

- Spinach salad with fresh raspberries, roasted almonds and crumbled feta cheese with a chicken breast or thigh, drizzled with olive oil and balsamic vinegar.
- Omelet with sun-dried tomatoes, spinach and feta cheese with two slices of natural turkey bacon.
- Cottage cheese, minced fresh ginger, pumpkin seeds, ground flaxseed and fresh berries with cinnamon.
- Ground dark chicken patties made with shredded onion and zucchini and a tablespoon of rolled oats, topped with grilled zucchini and organic sprouts, served with cut up carrots and cucumber with hummus and roasted artichoke hearts with olive oil.
- Carrot-ginger soup*, wild rice and lamb or veal chop.
- Wild salmon, steamed asparagus and black olive, cucumber and artichoke heart salad with olive oil, macadamia nut oil or hemp oil and herbs.
- Arugula salad or mixed greens with dried cranberries, maca damia nuts and diced turkey, drizzled with tahini (sesame seed butter).

- Quinoa and cucumber salad* with grilled tilapia with fresh rosemary and dill.
- Curried sweet potato and apple soup* with BBQ chicken breast topped with dandelion greens.
- Lentil soup* and slice of sprouted bread with hummus or walnut spread* and fresh spring cucumber.
- Two poached eggs over a bed of spinach and natural buffalo sausage.
- Plain organic yogurt, mixed berries, cinnamon, shredded coconut and a tablespoon of ground flaxseed, sunflower seeds or hemp seeds.
- Ezekiel wrap (health food stores) or nori wraps with lox (wild smoked salmon), spinach, shredded carrot, sprouts and artichoke hearts.
- Spinach salad with walnuts, strawberries and half a cup of chickpeas drizzled with tahini or hemp oil.
- Miso glazed salmon* with steamed broccoli with a teaspoon of ghee or butter and sautéed bok choy in tamari and garlic.
- Millet hot cereal with dollop of coconut milk, a tablespoon of sunflower seeds, fresh berries and ground flaxseed.

*These recipes can be found in *Putting it All Together: A Compilation of Healthy, Quick, Simple, Easy to Follow Recipes to Support You on Your Journey to Sound Nutrition* by Amy Bondar, available at the Hoffman Centre for Integrative Medicine.

"Dietary solutions need to be tailored to individuals because what works for one person may have no affect on another person, and may make a third person worse." –William Wolcott

Not too long ago, I am sure many of you had the opportunity to watch a show Oprah Winfrey hosted on anti-aging. Oprah interviewed a well-respected doctor who shared insights on how to slow the aging process and had some excellent health and nutrition tips. In fact it was nice to see Oprah focus on health and well being as opposed to her exhaustive topic of weight loss.

In one segment, the doctor shared a powerful tip: the importance of healthy bowel movements to health and well being. I could not agree more. Health begins in the colon. If you are not eliminating properly—excreting toxins and excess estrogens—you are putting your health at great risk. Constipation is serious. If any of you are experiencing it or are not eliminating at least one "banana shaped" stool once a day, come in and see me, especially if you are doing any form of detoxification. Many people just grab a fibre bulk when they are constipated, a foolish move because it just masks the problem. Your body has wisdom and it is risky to ignore. So don't hide out! Work with nutrition to detect what causes the slowing bowels, remedy the situation and support your colon properly. This is essential for optimum wellness.

Another segment of the show that I thought was excellent included a display of top food choices to slow down aging, prevent disease and maintain overall health. Oprah and the doctor made some valuable points, such as including healthy proteins at every meal and the importance of eating cruciferous vegetables. They promoted the best and safest mercury-free fish (wild salmon, sardines, tilapia, haddock and summer flounder). They touted berries as some of the greatest and most antioxidant rich fruits. Water and green tea were the beverages of choice and they even talked about the live food value of some whole grains such as quinoa, millet, buckwheat and steel cut oats versus the deadly white and refined grains and flours. And yes, they even agreed that a daily 24-oz cup of coffee, a glass of red wine and aspirin are important.

Now before you get all excited and run over to Starbucks, don't forget what I wrote about in Tip 7 and there is the one small thing Oprah forgot to mention: there is no one-size-fits-all approach to nutrition. Though the anti-aging show included some sound recommendations, they were very general and certainly could not take into account your individual health concerns, biochemistry or body types.

I strive to ensure that the nutritional programs I create for you are based on you, and you alone. So before you take Oprah's show, or a new magazine article or the DVD your friend gave you as "the" nutrition answer, consider that:

- Though the proteins are important, they are not all created equal in every body. Your metabolic type and Ayurvedic constitution determine which proteins are best and most balancing for you.
- The cruciferous vegetables (broccoli, broccoli sprouts, cauli flower, cabbage, kale, bok choy and Brussels sprouts) are incredibly important for liver detoxification and the prevention of breast cancer and osteoporosis. They are high in antioxidants. However, if you have a weakened thyroid, you must know that your body wants to eat these vegetables cooked or steamed ONLY. When eaten raw, the goitrogens in the cruciferous vegetables can block the production of the thyroid hormone.
- The recommendation of four servings a day of whole grains was also extremely general. That is too much unless you are

a carbohydrate metabolic type. If you have hypoglycemia, candidiasis, diabetes, obesity, fungus, parasites, sinusitis, compromised digestion, eczema, asthma, high blood pressure, high triglycerides or high cholesterol, you cannot eat that much grain and grain flour. Oprah's guest pointed out the importance of whole wheat and did not at the same time caution about gluten (protein of wheat, rye, spelt, barley, kamut) for the one in four people who are actually gluten intolerant. He also failed to mention that wheat spikes the blood sugars higher and faster than any other grain so for anybody wanting to slow the aging process, prevent or fight hypoglycemia, insulin resistance and Type II diabetes, to name a few, wheat should be avoided.

- And then there's the coffee. The doctor did say that coffee could have some protective properties. He also warned that it is a drug and does have side effects. If you are balanced and have no health concerns then perhaps a daily SMALL cup of coffee (less than 24 oz) won't hurt. If you have adrenal fatigue, high blood pressure, hypoglycemia, are a protein metabolic type, a vata dosha, or your sympathetic system is in over-drive (this is the case for most North Americans), coffee is more detrimental than beneficial to your health.

- As for the daily glass of red wine... Again, red wine is protective for some. Red wine does contain some antioxidants; at the same time, alcohol increases the risk of almost every form of cancer (except prostate and possibly bladder). If you have hormonal imbalances, a history of cancer in your family, obesity, or are doing a liver detoxification program, all alcohol—including red wine daily—is not ideal. Once in a while, a glass of red wine is fine, but on a daily basis it may be more of a risk factor than a protective factor.

And now for the aspirin a day…I leave this one to you. After all, it has been a standard recommendation for years. Personally, though, I won't put anything in my body every day that is made up of coal tar. That includes aspirin!

So the bottom line is this: Consider all those health options that you see on TV and read in books, but stop and ask yourself, "Did anyone consider if this is right for my body type?"

Chances are you already know the answer is no. So remember that it is your body, your nutritional lifestyle and your journey to optimum wellness.

One of the most misunderstood macronutrients are essential fatty acids (EFAs). Essential fats are required to produce every single hormone in the body, they feed and fuel the brain, they balance insulin levels, burn body fat, play an integral role in the health of your skin, nails and hair, they boost immunity and they can play a significant role in turning on or off inflammatory markers in the body.

I always talk about the power of foods, and essential fatty acids are a perfect example of how a food can significantly affect the health of your human body—positively or negatively. Pay careful attention to the types of fats you eat and the proportions in which you eat them. As Dr. Jeanne Wallace, an expert on the role fats play in the health of the human body, explains,

> This is because the fats we eat in our diet can be converted in the body (and in the brain) to a special type of hormone-like chemicals called prostaglandins. Some prostaglandins are beneficial, while other can be quite harmful and promote inflammation.[1]

Whether they are beneficial or harmful depends on the kinds and ratio of fatty acids ingested.

In order to prevent inflammation, the ratio of omega-3:6 must be 1:4. According to Dr. Ron Rosedale and Dr. Joseph Mercola, two leaders in metabolic medicine, the average ratio for North Americans is 1:25–50!!! This enormous fatty acid imbalance sets the stage for silent inflammation, chronic disease, accelerated aging and an ongoing state of less than optimal health.

To understand how we have become so imbalanced, it is important to know something about the kinds and sources of the fats we eat. There are three families of fats: omega-3, omega-6 and omega-9.

Omega-3 fats include those from flaxseed, flax oil hempseed, hemp oil, macadamia nut oil, fish and fish oils These are key players in turning off inflammation. That is why they are promoted in your nutritional and supplemental protocols. These oils go through an intricate biochemical breakdown before the body absorbs them in their anti-inflammatory form. The oils don't do this by themselves. The process requires mineral levels to be optimal. If you are deficient in minerals, you cannot break these fats down properly. The one exception to this rule is the fish oils. The fish oils automatically absorb into the body as anti-inflammatory prostaglandins without having to go through that biochemical breakdown process. This is why in most cases I promote the use of fish oils more than the other oils if you are deficient in essential fats.

Omega-6 fats come in two kinds: healthy fats and toxic fats. The healthy fats include lean animal protein, nuts, seeds, avocado, egg yolks, butter, evening primrose and borage oil. Focus on these healthy fats to make up your 1:4 ratio. The unhealthy, harmful and toxic omega-6 fats to stay away from include the high saturated fats found in grain-fed beef, vegetable oils (canola, margarine, soybean oil, corn oil, safflower, sunflower, peanut oil, cottonseed oil), partially hydrogenated fats, hydrogenated fats and trans-fats. You will find these toxic oils in all fast food, processed, packaged and manufactured foods such as commercial snack foods, baked goods, peanut butter, salad dressing, microwave popcorn, mayonnaise and so on. Beware of these fats! They are the precursors to turning on inflammation in your body.

Remember to eat only the kinds of omega-6 fats that are essential for health (as listed above). Amazingly enough, we have the power to convert them into beneficial prostaglandins (PGE1) or pro-inflammatory prostaglandins (PGE2). The way to make them beneficial as opposed to detrimental is to avoid sugar and refined carbohydrates. Dr. Jeanne Wallace explains, "Insulin secreted in response to glucose stimulates these oils to become harmful prostaglandins."[2] So a high sugar diet, erratic blood sugar and insulin levels and an influx of omega-6 fats guarantee you are stoking the inflammatory fires. No wonder North Americans are so inflamed!

Omega-9 fats (found in small amounts among many healthy fats, especially olive oil) are neutral and have no effect on inflammation.

It is important to note that essential fats are extremely therapeutic. In fact, they can act like a drug in the body. Supplement your diet with caution. Know that it is possible to overdo the good fats and even reverse the balanced ratio of 1:4. This is not safe either. So before you begin pouring in the fish oils, Udo's oil, omega-3: 6:9 blends and hemp oil, make sure you understand your own ratios of omega fats. Through your work with Dr. Hoffman, you will detect exactly which fats your individual biochemistry requires. If you are interested in knowing more about your essential fatty acid profile, Dr. Hoffman offers two laboratory tests. They will provide the information you need to be assured you are supplementing safely and accurately.

The nutritional lifestyle I customize for you is designed to rebalance your ratio of essential fatty acids to ensure that you are promoting the safe fats, eliminating the toxic and pro-inflammatory fats and eliminating insulin surging factors so you do not turn the potentially good fats against you.

You see my friends there is method to my madness!

I hold a vision for every one of my clients: I want to help you achieve optimum wellness through sound nutrition and that you will sustain optimum wellness in your life through a sound nutritional lifestyle. To that end, I have spent the past four years perfecting my nutritional program to ensure it is on the cutting-edge in achieving optimum wellness. I have begun compiling a list of benefits you can experience by using my 7 Steps to Sound Nutrition™ program and by embracing and implementing the wisdom from this book. I want to share this list with you with the hope that reading these actual benefits will inspire you to maintain your sound nutritional lifestyle indefinitely. My program includes at least the following benefits and attributes:

- Anti-inflammatory
- Anti-cancer and helps to fight existing cancers
- Anti-aging (slows the aging process)
- Prevents cardiovascular heart disease
- Supports detoxification
- Healthy, holistic and organic
- Combines Eastern, Western, traditional, scientific and holistic insights
- Advances optimum wellness
- Balances hormones
- Eases menopause symptoms
- Reverses PMS
- Promotes the healing and health of the colon
- Promotes liver health
- Prevents and reverses Syndrome X (high cholesterol, high triglycerides, high blood pressure, insulin resistance, obesity and Type II diabetes)

- Supports brain health
- Acknowledges biochemical individuality
- Customized for individual body types (Ayurvedic and metabolic typing)
- Promotes balance
- Supports and strengthens the endocrine system (thyroid and adrenals)
- Balances the autonomic nervous system
- Eliminates common food sensitivities
- Supports workouts and exercise
- Promotes natural and healthy weight loss and maintenance
- Increases energy and vitality
- Improves skin complexion
- Protects the health of the eyes
- Promotes hair and nail growth
- Prevents fibroids and endometriosis
- Promotes soulful nourishment by eating with intention and purpose
- Helps you to love your body for what it is, as it is
- Builds strength and confidence
- Moves you away from diet mentality
- Taps you in to nature's greatest medicine
- Builds in seasonal eating
- Strengthens the immune system
- Connects you and your body to nature and the environment
- Provides you the fuel to live the life you desire

Are you someone who has been struggling with weight for a long time and it doesn't seem to make a difference which program or diet you try because none of them seem to work? If so, I'd like to ask you to consider that your weight loss odyssey is bigger than will power, disciple, diligence and diet. It may not be about the food. Certainly it's more complicated than just knowing which foods to avoid and which foods to consume. If you have given your nutritional lifestyle a good run and your weight still stays stuck, then it is time to think beyond the physical realm and start working with the emotional body.

Consider the following questions:

- What am I holding on to?
- What do I not want to let go of?
- What is my body weight protecting me from?
- What am I swallowing?
- What am I having trouble digesting?
- What void am I filling?
- What hurt am I stuffing down?
- What comfort am I seeking from food that I feel I'm not getting elsewhere?
- Who am I putting a wall up from?
- Why do I not want to feel attractive or available?
- At what pivotal moment in my life did I start turning to food or gaining weight?
- How am I benefiting from being overweight?

If any of these questions resonate with you or you feel you need to explore further, then I urge you to come and do some emotional release work. Together, we explore emotional blocks that prevent you from reaching your weight loss and health goals. There are some emotional release tools and techniques that can help you to move and overcome those blocks and help you see that your weight struggle may indeed be about more than just the physical act of eating and may take more than simply following a nutritional plan. Your weight and relationship with food may actually root itself much deeper in the emotional body and perhaps even be so deep-rooted that you are not even conscious of it.

I highly recommend that you write these questions in a journal or at the back of this book in the designated section and take the time to answer them. You will be amazed at the unconscious thoughts you have been suppressing over the years. Perhaps this awakening and awareness will trigger a release and shedding of pounds.

Remember, your journey to optimum wellness looks at all possible reasons for disharmony, imbalance and discord within the body. Your nutritional challenges involve more than simply food and the physical and biochemical process of gaining and losing weight. To truly master your nutrition and optimize your health you will journey into the emotional, mental and spiritual realms as well.

"It's better to eat bad food with a good heart than good food with a bad heart." –Unknown

Every time you eat, you have the power to influence the way your body receives the food you are feeding it. The way you accept your food forwards or slows your nutritional mastery.

One of my goals as your Nutritional Consulting Practitioner is to teach and inspire you to maintain your nutritional lifestyles for a life-time. Throughout your life, there are definitely going to be numer-ous occasions where you indulge in foods that normally don't exist in your daily nutritional regimen. How you use the power of your thoughts with those foods matters on these occasions because they create the context for your next food choices.

For example, if you eat a piece of chocolate cake and tell your-self how bad it is for you, that you will gain five pounds by eating it and that you have no willpower, what is likely to happen? You will feel ill after eating it, gain the five pounds and burden yourself with feelings of guilt.

If you eat that same piece of chocolate cake and tell yourself that you would love to enjoy it, an occasional indulgence serves body and soul, and that you would love to reward yourself because you have been eating so clean all week, what is likely to happen? You will accept that piece of cake with joy. You will feel completely satis-fied, fulfilled and know you've nourished your soul.

When I am conducting your Comprehensive Nutritional Intake, I always ask you what your highest values are. The purpose is to help you begin to link your nutritional goals to the things that mean the most to you in your life. It is this link—not the "food" itself—that is behind your nutritional program success. So from the beginning, you know your purpose in prioritizing and maintaining your nutri-tional program for a lifetime.

For example, if family is your highest value, you are at a family celebration and there is a piece of chocolate cake in front of you. Ask yourself, "How will eating this piece of cake support my family?" If it will add to your enjoyment with family, make you feel good for treating yourself to that cake, if it is in good spirits and fun, it's likely that piece of cake will have no ill effects on your body.

If however, you are bored, sitting and watching television, upset or angry about something and you start thinking about that piece of chocolate cake, ask yourself, "How will eating this piece of cake support my family?" If your family is not around, if you know you will feel guilty for having eaten it and later will lash out at your family for no other reason but frustration with yourself for eating the cake, or you know you will keep your partner up all night with indigestion because you ate it, then eating that cake does not support your highest value and your body would likely receive it with ill effects.

These examples show how important it is to know your highest values and to link both daily eating and occasional indulgence choices to those values. At every moment of making a food choice, you have the opportunity to dictate the way in which your body accepts or rejects food. Before you choose whether to indulge or not, link your potential indulgences to your highest values. If you are actually going to go for the pleasure, at least have purpose in doing so.

a few more recipes...

Trying a new recipe is always a great way to add variety and enjoyment to your nutritional lifestyle. The recipes below are all excellent for the end of our wet spring season. Enjoy!

cauliflower-spinach toss

1 lb spinach
½ medium-size head cauliflower, broken into florets, and then cut into ½-inch thick slices
1 large avocado
6 tbsp extra virgin olive oil
3 tbsp freshly squeezed lemon juice
1 large clove garlic, minced or pressed
½ tsp each Celtic sea salt, mustard powder and dried basil
½ tsp pepper
Dash of ground nutmeg
½ cup pine nuts or slivered almonds

1   Discard tough stems from spinach. Plunge leaves into cold water to clean; lift out, pat dry and tear into bite-size pieces. Place in a bowl and add cauliflower.
2   Pit, peel and slice avocado. Dip avocado slices in lemon juice to coat, then add to spinach and cauliflower.
3   Combine olive oil, lemon juice, garlic salt, mustard, basil, pepper and nutmeg; blend well. Pour over salad; add nuts and gently mix to coat thoroughly.

artichoke and asparagus soup

1 16-oz can artichoke hearts
1 bunch asparagus, cut up
1 tbsp butter

1 med shallot, chopped
2 green onions, green and white parts, sliced
1 can water chestnuts, sliced
1 tsp Celtic sea salt
1 tbsp fresh tarragon leaves or 1 ½ tsp dried
½ cup macadamia nut butter or cashew butter
3 cups vegetables stock or water
10 sprigs fresh watercress, broken

1   Pour liquid from artichoke hearts in saucepan. Chop artichokes
    coarsely and set aside.
2   Into saucepan add butter, chopped shallot or green onion and
    asparagus. Simmer gently for 4–5 minutes until asparagus is
    fork tender.
3   Add artichokes, chestnuts, vegetable seasoning and tarragon.
    Heat through.
4   Add 2 cups water or vegetable stock to vegetables. Then stir
    1 cup of remaining stock gradually to nut butter until smooth,
    then carefully stir into soup. Stir soup frequently while heating
    over medium low heat until mixture is heated through. Do not let
    the soup boil.

cuban style fish

4 6-oz fillets of tilapia, halibut, sea bass or other firm white fish
1 tsp lime zest (from organic lime)
2 tbsp freshly squeezed lime juice
2 cloves garlic, chopped
2 tbsp chopped fresh cilantro
2 tbsp chopped fresh basil
½ tsp red pepper flakes
Celtic sea salt to taste
2 tbsp extra virgin olive oil

1. Combine lime zest and juice, garlic, cilantro, basil, red pepper flakes, salt and olive oil.
2. Place fish in an ovenproof baking dish and coat with marinade. Marinate for 30 minutes.
3. Preheat oven to 350°F.
4. Bake fish for 15–20 minutes or until juices are clear.

walnut spread

1 cup garbanzo beans (chickpeas)
½ cup chopped walnuts
½ cup basil leaves
2 tbsp olive oil
2–3 tsp lemon juice
Dash salt and pepper

1. Drain beans and reserve liquid.
2. In blender or food processor, combine beans with 2 tbsp bean liquid and remaining ingredients.
3. Cover and blend until smooth. Add additional liquid as needed and scrape sides of bowl periodically.
4. Store in refrigerator and use as a dip for raw vegetables. Use within 5 days.

All recipes can be found in: *Putting It All Together: A Compilation of Healthy, Quick, Simple, Easy-to-Follow Recipes to Support You on Your Journey to Sound Nutrition* by Amy Bondar. It really is an excellent resource to ensure your nutritional journey is a tasty one!

"When your vegetables [and fruits] are grown organically, you are assured that your food is wholesome, that you are supporting an environmentally conscious farmer, that you are helping protect all the creatures in the ecosystem, and that you are protecting the land through wise and sustainable practices." –Jeff Cox

It is time again to be present with another season, time to transition our diets for summer's balancing foods. If you have been eating seasonally, in the last few months, you have cleansed your liver, burned off excess winter body fat, moved away from a heavy winter diet to one that is focused on bitter spring foods and successfully planted your garden. Now it is time to watch what you planted flourish.

Summer brings qualities of growth, fulfillment, high energy, vibrancy, rejuvenation and good times. It is important in this season to nourish our bodies with lots of light, fresh, magnetic-rich and wholesome fuel.

The element of summer is fire, so rid the diet of foods that create too much heat in the body. This is especially important for all those pitta types (see Tip 46), who can easily get aggravated, imbalanced and "fired-up" when overheated. Eliminating refined foods, black tea, coffee, alcohol, tobacco, excess red meat, spicy and salty foods, dairy products and fatty foods will prevent the body from becoming too heated during the summer season.

The key is healthy summer eating; focus on cooling, light and high energy foods that both fuel us through the long days and support the increased activity and exercise we are enjoying. The body in summer naturally gravitates to more fruits, vegetables, salads, lots of water and fewer and lighter meats, such as chicken and fish.

In fact, in the summer months a higher carbohydrate diet evolves naturally. This is the time when we consume far more fruits and vegetables than any other time of the year. According to John Douillard in *The 3-Season Diet:*

> …The low-fat spring harvest annually resets the body's ability to metabolize fat as fuel, forcing the body to burn its own fat for energy. When the high-energy, high carb summer harvest arrives, the body's baseline energy supply has already been set from the fat-burning of spring, preventing the high-sugar foods of summer from causing blood sugar highs and lows.[1]

This is the beauty of eating with the seasons. Our body transitions to what Mother Nature provides for us. The foods available to us in every season provide a purpose and play out biochemical roles in our bodies. We ignore at our own peril the innate intelligence of nature and what it has to offer. The more we connect with the seasons and eat what grows and subsists in nature the easier and more natural it is to achieve and maintain optimum wellness (i.e. balance) throughout the entire year.

The following is a list of the most balancing fruits and vegetables, to emphasize at this time of year.

june

- Asparagus
- Beets
- Carrots
- Cherries
- English peas
- Green peppers
- Lettuce
- New potatoes

- Radishes
- Spinach

july

- Apricots
- Blackberries
- Blueberries
- Carrots
- Cherries
- Field tomatoes
- Green peppers
- Lettuce
- Peaches
- Peas
- Plums
- Raspberries
- Spinach
- Strawberries
- Sweet onions

At every seasonal shift I invite you to come in for a nutritional session to fine-tune your diet, learn how to make seasonal food choices, create variety and ensure balance in the body. The foods listed above are only a general list and you want to be certain you are eating the best seasonal offerings for your unique Ayurvedic dosha, metabolic type and specific conditions. If you would love to stay as healthy and balanced as you can throughout the year, check in soon so your body can gain the most from your food choices this season.

favorite summer recipes

While savoring every bite of my crisp, sweet and luscious cherries last night, I found myself thinking how wonderful it is to be so connected to the glorious bounty that Mother Nature brings forth every season. I burst with energy when the seasons change, because it is a chance for me to switch up my diet, create more variety, listen to and learn what my body craves for wellness. Which nutrients? From what fruits and vegetables? What new foods or seasonal favorites will I discover at markets and health food stores?

This week it is my pleasure to share some summer favorites with you. Enjoy!

amy's homemade granola

1 cup organic 100% oats (long cooking)
½ cup organic ground flaxseed
½ cup organic hemp seed
½ cup organic raw, unsalted almonds
½ cup organic raisins
½ cup shredded, organic non-GMO, unsweetened coconut

1   In a large glass jar or a mixing bowl with a lid combine all of the ingredients.
2   Each night take ½ cup granola and put it into a bowl.
3   Fill the bowl with spring water, until water just covers the ingredients. Let soak overnight to release enzymes to make it easy to digest.
4   In the morning enjoy a bowl of granola with fresh raspberries and organic yogurt.

gazpacho soup

1 large English cucumber, diced
½ cup green pepper, diced
1 small onion (sweet—Wala Wala), diced
2 tsp fresh garlic
2 28-oz can whole tomatoes (or 1 can and 4–5 large fresh tomatoes, diced)
1 can Clamato juice
2 tsp fresh lemon juice
Celtic sea salt and pepper to taste
2 tbsp fresh parsley
2 tbsp fresh Cilantro

1 In a large pot combine the ingredients.
2 Purée ingredients in a food processor.
3 Chill in the refrigerator for 3 hours. Enjoy this gazpacho with a chicken breast or fresh tilapia.

bbq and fresh summer vegetables

In the summer evenings I love to barbecue any protein (fish, chicken pieces, steaks, buffalo burgers and so on) and accompany it with an array of flavorful and colorful vegetables. Here are some favorites:

- BBQ chicken or turkey breast served with lightly steamed (5–7 minutes) green beans with a teaspoon of ghee and raw sweet orange pepper slices with walnut spread
- BBQ salmon or tilapia accompanied by steamed asparagus (5–7 minutes) topped with a teaspoon of ghee, and Israeli salad (cucumber, tomato and black olives) with olive oil, oregano and dill

- BBQ chicken thighs, legs and wings along with steamed broccoli and a salad of spinach, shredded carrot and raspberries drizzled with olive oil

Note that there is no need to douse the meat with high-sugar, preservative-rich, nutrition-poor BBQ sauce. Instead, just use some fresh herbs, spices and lemon juice for a great light and healthy taste or use Dr. Mercola's Cornell BBQ Sauce recipe from Tip 47.

snacks

- It's all about the low-glycemic fresh fruits (cherries, peaches, nectarines, plums, blueberries, raspberries and so on). Enjoy them alone or with some pumpkin seeds.
- It's all about the fresh vegetables too—garden peas, carrots, cucumber and sweet orange peppers with hummus.

So, my friends, now you have peered into my summer diet and perhaps you can see the kaleidoscope of foods and the energy and vitality sound nutrition and healthy seasonal eating has to offer. The approach I describe is designed specifically for my body type. To fine tune your own summer selections, please contact me soon. You and your body will be glad you did!

Summer is the time when most of us find ourselves more physically active than at any other time of year. Because exercise and nutrition go hand in hand, knowing how to fuel your workouts and nourish post-exercise ensures that your body repairs and rejuvenates itself optimally. As Dr. Michael Colgan states in *Optimum Sports Nutrition,* "...nutrition is a magic bullet that will help you more than you ever dreamed to achieve your athletic goals."[1]

The more active you are the more nutrients you need to sustain physical performance. If you work out regularly, eat small frequent meals throughout the day (every three–four hours). This will enable you to maximize body fat loss, build muscle mass and maximize energy storage for your next workout.

What you fuel your body with at each one of those small meals impacts what you can achieve. The power of foods influences your hormones; for optimum performance, you need to consider three specific hormones: insulin, serotonin and dopamine.

insulin

The key to burning body fat, building muscle mass and maximizing your athletic performance is to keep your insulin levels stable. Many athletes are used to "carbo-loading." This can be unwise. Overeating carbohydrates (especially high glycemic carbohydrates such as white rice, pasta, floured breads and sugar) results in too much glucose entering into the bloodstream at one time. This elevates your insulin levels. Your body then burns muscle mass instead of body fat and stores fat instead of muscle mass. So eat to keep insulin levels stable!

serotonin

Eating too much glucose and/or carbohydrates prior to a workout triggers a release of the hormone serotonin. Serotonin "dulls" the nervous system. It limits the amount of muscle you can contract which will then limit your energy, endurance and performance.

dopamine

Dopamine, on the other hand, will maximize your muscle endurance resulting in running harder, faster and longer. The focus then is to release dopamine by eating protein before a workout. Some of the highest dopamine rich foods include: chicken, turkey, game meat, walnuts and cottage cheese. Eating more protein and less glucose two hours before your workout is the way to manipulate the synergy of serotonin and dopamine.

To balance insulin, serotonin and dopamine always combine your carbohydrates with protein and essential fats. Choose fibrous carbohydrates—fruits, vegetables and minimal gluten-free whole grains (oats, quinoa, brown rice, wild rice, millet, sprouted breads, buckwheat and amaranth). This combination will prevent spikes in blood sugars and the release of too much serotonin and you will enjoy increased energy, endurance and performance.

There is a point at which carbohydrate consumption in your body exceeds the level at which it can be used for energy or stored as body fat. Over a three–four hour period, women can use only 25 grams of carbohydrates (½ cup rice or a piece of sprouted bread) and men can use only 50 grams of carbohydrates (1 cup rice or two pieces of sprouted bread). Any more than that can tip the balance of the three hormones. Too low a carbohydrate intake can also hinder your performance, so it becomes important to find and use your personal fuel mix.

Remember to nourish your body post-workout, too! This will provide you with the nutrients for muscle repair and growth and the energy to store for your next workout. A protein shake is always an excellent and convenient fuel mix within 30 minutes of a workout. A protein shake provides the perfect combination of protein, essential fats and glucose. Ensure you eat a main meal one and a half to two hours after that. Here is an ideal workout fuel plan:

pre-workout
breakfast
½ cup of cottage cheese
A tablespoon of ground flaxseed
Fresh berries

post-workout
Protein shake (whey, berries, half a banana, water and hemp oil)

lunch
Spinach salad
Turkey breast or chicken thigh
A tablespoon of olive oil

snack
3–4 tablespoons of walnuts
Apple or pear

dinner
Wild salmon or game meat
1 cup wild rice or quinoa (men)
½ cup wild rice or quinoa (women)
Steamed asparagus with teaspoon ghee or butter
Salad with olive oil

Remember every body is different. Finding your personal fuel mix based on your metabolic type is the best way to ensure you are giving your body the specific nutrients it needs. Your body knows how to perform optimally when it has the right fuel. If you are lacking energy, strength and endurance during your workouts you know you are not hitting your fuel mix. At that realization please come in to see me to fine-tune your diet so you can gain the results you are working to achieve.

*Some of the above information is from, "The Science of Endurance Nutrition," a video by Lars Gustafson.

The cruciferous vegetables are a family of vegetables that I strongly emphasize as part of your nutritional lifestyle. Bok choy, broccoli, broccoli sprouts, Brussels sprouts, cabbage, cauliflower, kale, collard greens, watercress, arugula, kohlrabi and mustard greens are part of the Brassica or 'cabbage' family and are some of the most important vegetables you can eat to optimize health.

For those of you who grow some of these vegetables in your own garden, you can see that they emit great power, precision, strength and beauty. These vegetables are so powerful that they seem truly to speak of healing.

Study after study has shown that the greater amount of cruciferous vegetables eaten, the more cancer rates decline. This is especially true for lung cancer, gastrointestinal cancers and hormonal dependant cancers such as breast and prostate. Adding 500 grams of broccoli or other cruciferous vegetables a day (approximately 2 ½ cups) to your sound nutritional lifestyles can speak volumes both in the prevention of cancer and in fighting an existing cancer.

Eating cruciferous vegetables is also one of the most profound things you can do to support detoxification because these vegetables activate phase II liver detoxification. This fact is especially important for people who have high levels of estrogen (postmenopausal women, those with PMS, those with breast or prostate cancer, etc.) in their bodies. According to Dr. Robert Rountree, an expert on the role Brassica vegetables play in detoxification and health, "It's not the estrogen that's the problem. It's what the liver does with the estrogen that's important."[1] So the more cruciferous vegetables you eat, the better your liver can process and wipe out the "bad" estrogen and promote the "good" estrogen. This may be why these vegetables are so successful in cutting the risk of hormone dependant cancers.

Cruciferous vegetables are also promoted for all of you who have arthritis, osteoporosis and other muscular-skeletal conditions as they are rich in calcium, vitamin K and sulfur—three nutrients needed for healthy muscles, joints and bones. Sulfur also plays a significant role in protecting against fungi, bacteria and parasites, so for compromised digestion, these vegetables can also play a healing role.

Consider as well the amazing antioxidant effects of a diet high in cruciferous vegetables. They fight chemical carcinogens and prevent damage to DNA. Numerous in-vitro and animal studies show that they stop the growth of cancer cells. A diet high in antioxidants (supplied by cruciferous vegetables) is the best way to reverse inflammation (and hence prevent all types of chronic disease) and slow the aging process.

It is best to eat these vegetables raw (chew well!), because they stay in your bloodstream longer than if they were cooked. This means the nutritive compounds will have a prolonged effect in the body. Juicing these vegetables is also ideal.

I have cautioned against eating these vegetables raw if you have low thyroid function, because naturally occurring goitrogens in these foods can hinder the production of the thyroid hormone. Recently, however, research reported in two different seminars, both concluded that it is not yet clear how goitrogens affect the thyroid hormone and how much it would actually take to have an adverse affect. It appears you would have to eat several pounds of raw crucifers a day to make a difference. So though I have cautioned it in previous tips, know that you are likely fine if you eating cruciferous vegetables raw in moderation.

It is important to note that the flavanoids in these vegetables are easily destroyed by certain cooking methods:

- Microwaving: 97% destroyed
- Boiling: 66% destroyed
- Steaming (5–7 minutes): Minimal loss

So, for maximum nutritive power and healing potential eat the cruciferous vegetables raw, juiced or lightly steamed.

I have always advocated that food can be our greatest medicine and weapon against chronic disease and I am not alone. The first recorded description of the power of cruciferous vegetables in particular is from Cato in Rome, 234–149 BC: "If a cancerous ulcer appears upon the breast, apply a crushed cabbage leaf and it will make it well." There is no question that we should all focus on adding more of these vegetables to our diet. I recommend eating three to four cups of vegetables a day and I urge you to ensure that two of those cups come from the cruciferous family.

summer herbs & spices

"Food is the chief of all things. It is therefore said to be medicine for all diseases of the body." –Taittiraya Upanishad

Herbs and spices, spices and herbs—a fantastic addition to your nutritional lifestyle. They offer color, variety, distinct taste, inviting aromas and powerful medicinal effects. In summer, you may enjoy the herbs and spices growing in your garden or find yourself more interested in those you see at the markets and health food stores. Still, you may not be aware of just how much nutritional benefit accompanies the delight to the senses of herbs and spices. So this nutritional tip is dedicated to sharing some of the secrets hidden within some of nature's greatest gems.

parsley

- Reduces blood pressure
- Diuretic (helpful to ease bloating before women's periods)
- Strengthens the digestive system
- Aids in metabolism
- Purifies the blood and accelerates the excretion of toxins
- Eases bloating, stomach cramps and nausea
- High in iron, making it a great blood tonic
- Relieves arthritic symptoms
- Helps support the liver and kidney

chives

- High in vitamin C, folic acid and potassium
- Eases stomach stress
- Protects against heart disease and stroke
- Aids in the digestion of fat
- Stimulates the appetite and promote good digestion

- Prevents bad breath
- Clears sinuses

dill

- Good for stomach and intestinal problems
- Improves mild insomnia
- Eases flatulence and heart burn
- Dill tea is a remedy for hiccups
- Supports liver and gallbladder
- Dill tea can also stimulate milk production for nursing mothers and soothe colic in babies

cilantro

- Stimulates appetite and improves digestion
- Pulls heavy metals out of the body
- Good for migraines

basil

- Aids in digestion by increasing saliva and bile flow
- Antispasmodic (eases flatulence, nausea, motion sickness and bronchial spasms)
- Stimulates the cilia in the nose, helping to clear the nasal passageways
- Protects against flies and mosquitoes, making it a good choice to keep in your garden

tarragon

- Treats digestive complaints and stimulates the appetite
- Beneficial for tooth aches
- Stimulates the production of bile which is beneficial for the gallbladder and digestion of fats

- May promote menstruation, fight fatigue and calm the nervous system
- Helps fight parasites

hyssop

- Relieves the irritations of colds and allergies (coughs, congestion and sore throats)
- Stimulates the digestive juices to break down foods
- Antiseptic—good for skin conditions or cold sores

dandelion

- Stimulates digestive secretions
- Rids liver and gallbladder of waste products
- Helps body eliminate toxins through the skin making it beneficial for acne, eczema and psoriasis
- High in potassium making it an excellent diuretic, helping alleviate fluid retention

rosemary

- Helps bloating and cramps
- Stimulates the appetite and promotes digestion
- Uplifts and revitalizes

One of the common themes amongst all these herbs and spices is that they are powerful digestive aids. Adding any of the above to your meals or steeping them as teas can greatly enhance your digestion. They are also a wonderful way to create variety in your meals, salads and soups.

There is beauty, history and healing in all herbs and spices. So this summer take advantage of their abundance. Experiment and add a powerful new zing to your nutritional lifestyle.

Metabolic typing is one of the most important steps in my 7 Steps to Sound Nutrition™ program. In fact, it is the pivotal piece that frees you to determine your unique nutritional needs. Your body is designed to be healthy. Every cell in the body is programmed for health. The key is to ensure you provide your body with the building blocks (genetic requirements) it needs to function optimally.

Metabolic typing is about fueling the autonomic nervous system (ANS)—the grand regulator of every metabolic process in the human body. The ANS controls all unconscious life-sustaining functions. It serves you when you are unaware and serves you brilliantly when you eat according to your metabolic type. When you eat right for your metabolic type, you maximize energy and efficiency for every system in the body.

Since each cell in the body knows what to do when given the right foods and nutrients, metabolic typing provides the foundation to reverse degenerative disease or prevent disease from occurring. William Wolcott, one of the pioneers of metabolic typing states,

> Metabolic Typing is geared toward building health by correcting the patterns of biochemical imbalance that underlie, or are at the root of, chronic health problems.[1]

As you may now know, my nutritional practice is based on biochemical individuality. I have always counseled that there is no one-size-fits-all approach to nutrition. That is the beauty of a system like metabolic typing (and Ayurvedic nutrition). Metabolic typing is the science that dictates the response your body will have to certain foods and nutrients. It allows you to fine tune nutritional needs and choices based on inherent and individual body make-up. As Wolcott explains,

Even if you consume the highest quality and most healthful foods and supplements it's entirely possible that you are mal-nourished if those specific foods and nutrients don't match your Metabolic Type.[2]

When determining your metabolic type we need to understand the two branches to the ANS—the parasympathetic branch (rest and digest) and the sympathetic branch (fight or flight). In most people one branch of the system dominates, and the other system is weaker. The ANS is out of balance. All metabolic imbalances can be corrected by using food to strengthen the weaker side of the ANS. Our symptoms are tied to whether our sympathetic or para-sympathetic system is more dominant. The key is to determine the dominant side and then manipulate the diet to build up the weaker or more recessive side.

When you eat according to your metabolic type your body moves to a state of balance, offering greater emotional poise, mental clarity, peaceful energy, improved well being, better sleep, increased energy, normalization of body weight, alleviation of cravings and regeneration and repair of cells. You will also have a greater sense of certainty as to what foods and what ratios of foods work best for your individual body. It truly takes the guesswork out of eating.

It takes energy to reverse degenerative disease and achieve optimum wellness. For example, if you are doing mercury detoxi-fication, which demands a great deal of energy, eating right for your metabolic type will provide your cells with that energy. If you have multiple sclerosis, your goal is to repair and regenerate cells; eating right for your metabolic type will provide cells with the energy needed to do that. If you have quit smoking, your cells need to regenerate, but they can only do so if you provide them with the right building blocks. Again, eating according to your metabolic type will do just that.

The efficiency of your body to heal or become well depends on the energy or quality of fuel you give it. Your body's unique set of cells, tissues, glands, organs and systems all require specific energy and you can determine your specific energy requirements by understanding your unique metabolic type.

Metabolic typing is believed to be the future of medicine. You cannot build your foundation for health, master your nutritional lifestyle or optimize results without knowing, understanding and fueling your metabolic type.

As you journey through the Hoffman Centre for Integrative Medicine, you are looking at more than just your physical body to explain why you are feeling the way you are. Each level of Dr. Bruce Hoffman's 7 Levels of Healing™ model peels another layer, offers new insight and provides you with healing modalities and therapies to help resolve imbalances.

Sound nutrition can be applied to each of the 7 Levels of Healing™. For those who have not yet been through this evolutionary model, the seventy-five nutrition tips in this book actually guide you through those seven levels. These tips take you from the first level of understanding how toxins in your food can affect your health, all the way to the seventh level in which spiritual connection with the power of foods helps you create the life you desire. The purpose of these tips is to inspire, educate and motivate you to realize that sound nutrition goes far beyond the physical. If you truly embrace it, sound nutrition will guide and support you on your journey to optimum wellness.

What follows is a blueprint of how nutrition fits into the 7 Levels of Healing™. It is a reminder to look more deeply into what your food intake can offer you, and a reminder to tap into nutrition at every level of healing. It is intended to help you truly see that your nutritional lifestyle is capable of initiating healing through your physical body and beyond.

level one: the extended body

Toxicology is one of the first places we look for possible explanations for your symptoms, illnesses and imbalances. It has been estimated that over 50,000 toxic chemicals are in commercial use today. We know that many diseases actually are environmental diseases, meaning they have been caused by exposure to toxins in our environment. We live in an extremely toxic world and without proper nutrition and regular detoxification, our bodies become overburdened. As a result we manifest with symptoms that cannot yet be explained.

There is no question that our nutritional intake can add to that toxic burden. We know that pesticides, herbicides and other chemicals that are sprayed on foods damage our health. Plastics in which we store our food or from which we drink water can leach xenoestrogens into our bodies and increase our risk of certain cancers. Using Teflon and aluminum cookware adds more heavy metal exposure to our bodies. Hormones, antibiotics and genetically modified foods also affect our health negatively. If we do not wash our foods properly we can be host for many parasites and bacterial infections. Other foods carry mycotoxins (fungal toxins) than can overburden our bodies. The list goes on, but the point of this tip is not to paint a bleak picture. It is to help you see that through better nutrition choices you can lessen the toxic load in your body and increase your own health and wellness.

Choosing to eat organic produce and meats, foods that grow and subsist in nature, non-GMO foods, using glass containers to store foods, drinking from Nalgene water bottles, using ceramic cookware, purchasing local produce over exported produce and avoiding processed, packaged, manufactured foods are all excellent and easy to adopt nutritional tips that you can use to help peel that first layer and move you closer to a state of wellness.

level two: the physical body

Understanding your body's biochemistry is one of the most fascinating opportunities you will have at the Hoffman Centre for Integrative Medicine. Your physical body is your foundation and sound nutrition and therapeutic foods (supplements) are the key players in ensuring that the foundation is operating efficiently and optimally.

Micronutrient (vitamins and minerals) and macronutrient (proteins, essential fats, carbohydrates and water) deficiencies can induce DNA damage and disease expression. Dr. Hoffman intricately puts together your body's biochemical puzzle and through extensive laboratory work, testing and insight, he detects the pieces of that puzzle that are missing, deficient or in need of support.

Your nutritional program and comprehensive nutritional intake and analyses are designed to rebuild and strengthen your foundation and to fill in those missing pieces. Supplements are added because your body's detoxification mechanisms are dependant on proteins, essential fats and antioxidants. Food sensitivities and allergies are eliminated because they impede the body's ability to heal. Understanding your individual body type (Ayurvedic dosha and metabolic type) is pivotal in creating the balance in your foundation; it is this balance that fuels your cells, tissues, organs, glands and systems. Calming your sympathetic system (stress response) with the power of foods is also essential for the healing process to be initiated. Without all these pieces in place, your body can run only sub-optimally. The power of foods is incredible and many of you have seen that the slightest eliminations, additions and adjustments to your diets make a tremendous difference in how you feel and in affecting and altering your biochemistry.

level three: the electromagnetic body

Here is where we speak of energy. Food is one of our greatest suppliers of vital energy, prana, life force or chi. When you eat whole, live, magnetic-rich food, your cells vibrate with that same energy. Contrast that with the energy of foods you eat that are processed in factories, stripped of nutrients or have a long shelf life. These dead foods offer no vitality; as a result your cells vibrate at a very dull level. You can feel this energy shift at grocery stores. Large commercial grocery stores have a very different kind of energy than that of health food stores or farmer's markets.

Organic vegetable juicing can be introduced at this level to help increase the live magnetic energy you can provide your cellular body. It has been said that organic foods have more light energy than non-organic foods because there is more chlorophyll (oxygen) trapped into the light of these foods. It is also at this level that we detect food sensitivities so that we can remove any possible factors that may be blocking, weakening or stressing the energy circuits in the body.

We also recommend avoiding microwaving as it destroys all live enzymes, nutrients and light in food. Another incredibly important energetic principle to tap into is eating in a parasympathetic state, eating with intention, connection and awareness as these all increase the absorption of nutrients, allowing for more energy.

Even eating seasonally allows us to tap into greater energies beyond our physical bodies. When we tap into the energetic cycles of Mother Nature and naturally change our food choices with the seasons, we maintain energetic balance throughout the year. So, you can see that even at the energetic level, your nutritional choices have great influence in your healing process.

level four: the emotional body

There is no question that our emotions influence our biochemistry and at the Hoffman Centre for Integrative Medicine we believe tapping into the emotional field and uncovering and transcending emotional blocks is key to your healing process. Understanding your emotional connection and dependency on food can be one of the most challenging pieces to overcome on your journey to optimum wellness.

Here is where working with Steve Harvey and using the Demartini Method® (also known as the Quantum Collapse Process®) can offer great insight and help you transcend emotional dependency on food. Emotional Freedom Technique and The Demartini Method® are profound modalities that can offer insights and practical tools to prevent you from letting your emotions run your food choices.

Food also offers us positive feelings, memories and experiences and is used for many as a means for celebration, a purpose to gather with friends or just treat ourselves to the simple pleasures we desire the most.

level five: the intellectual body

The intellectual body is where beliefs and ego constructs can affect food choices. This is where values come into play. Rationally, we all know we should eat well, but reason and logic take us only so far. We need purpose to maintain our nutritional lifestyle. In Step One of my 7 Steps to Sound Nutrition™ program I always ask about highest values because when you can link your nutritional goals to the things that matter the most to you in your life, you have purpose to make nutrition of more importance to you, so you maintain your programs at greater ease.

This is where I also help you move away from diet mentality and see that your food choices are about more than just losing weight, they are about creating health. We look at the importance of eating quality over quantity (fat grams, calories and carbs). It is here where we also use the Demartini Method® to teach you to love your body for what it is as it is rather than attach to a fantasy of looking a certain way.

Often, our beliefs around food can be limiting to our healing potential but again, by using the Demartini Method® and Emotional Freedom Technique with Steve Harvey you can shift the way you view food and continue forward on your journey toward optimum wellness.

When you are in tune with your soul body you are connected to your life's purpose. This is when you use food for energetic fuel and mental and spiritual clarity to fulfill all that you desire in life. This is when you become truly connected to how foods make you feel and make your food choices based on what will keep your Ayurvedic dosha and metabolic body type in balance.

It is here that you may create a sacred eating space (see Tip 71), say mantras while eating to increase the efficacy of the foods within the body, and feel grateful for the food you are eating, as you know it is the source of light and energy for you.

level seven: the spiritual body

Surrendering to a greater intelligence of the universe, understanding that the body knows how to heal itself when given the right nutrients, being humbled to the fact that the body will always be in a state of build and destroy, health and disease, balance and imbalance, trusting that nature provides us all we need to heal, loving our bodies for what they are as they are, being truly grateful and seeing the order in everything, is when you have awakened to the spiritual body.

It can be said that food offers us all we need; food is everything. It stimulates the senses, tantalizes the mind and connects us to our soul and spirit. It is our prana, our life force. It is light and love. When you use food in this manner you have truly made a shift in consciousness.

healing recipes

"Drugs work, no doubt about it. But optimum nutrition works equally as well and has no downside, neither for health nor for the human spirit." –Dr. Michael Colgan

"Let food be thy medicine and thy medicine be thy food." Hippocrates, considered by many as the founder of modern medicine, wrote this nearly 2300 years ago. Those of you who follow my nutritional program have experienced just how powerful food truly can be in achieving your health goals.

Nature provides the foods and herbs we need for whatever may ail us. Following are some recipes that can be used in times when the body needs to be strengthened, tended to and healed.

bieler broth[1]

This broth is highly recommended for those under stress or with adrenal fatigue. The broth provides the perfect balance of sodium and potassium to overworked organs and glands, especially the sodium-loving adrenal glands (ever wonder why you crave salt when stressed?) This broth restores energy and can be used for overall health.

4 medium squash (zucchini, yellow or summer) washed, ends removed and sliced
1 lb string beans, ends removed
2 bunches parsley, stems removed
Fresh herbs, such as thyme or tarragon, tied together with a string
1 quart filtered water
Whey (optional)

1   Place water, vegetables and herbs in a pot. Bring to a boil, skim, lower heat and simmer, covered, for 30 minutes.

2 Remove herbs.
3 Vegetables may be eaten whole with cooking water, or blended into a thick soup with a handheld blender. One tablespoon of whey can be added to each cup of soup—this maximizes the absorption of potassium and other minerals.

hijiki salad[2]

Hijiki is seaweed rich in calcium, iron, iodine and B vitamins. It helps detoxify the body, normalizes blood sugars, aids in weight loss, balances hormones, supports the thyroid and soothes nerves.

1 cup hijiki, soaked and cut
1 tsp oil or ½ cup water
2 tbsp umeboshi vinegar, rice vinegar or lemon juice
1 carrot, grated
½ cup onion, chopped
Sea salt to taste

1 Sauté hijiki in oil 20–30 minutes or cook in water. Allow to cool.
2 Mix all ingredients together and serve on mixed greens.

chicken soup

Chicken broth is great for whatever ails you. It is extremely beneficial for colds, flu, fatigue, soulful nourishment and digestive discomfort. There are many homemade chicken soup recipes available, so if not this one, others will do.

1 ½ gallons water
Bones, feet and other parts from 2 chickens
2 carrots
2 celery stalks
3 tbsp each of parsley and cilantro

2-inch piece of ginger

½ celery root

2 red potatoes

5 garlic cloves

1 onion

1 turnip.

3–4 tbsp any vinegar of your choice

1–2 tbsp Celtic sea salt

1   Cut and quarter all veggies into 2–3 inch pieces.
2   Put all ingredients in large soup pot. Bring to boil and simmer for 6–15 hours.
3   Let cool, strain and store broth in fridge. Discard all of the veggies and bones.

potassium broth[3]

This is a fantastic broth for those who need to support the liver, rejuvenate from chemotherapy or for women who are recovering from childbirth.

4 potatoes, organic, well scrubbed

3 carrots, peeled and chopped

4 celery sticks, chopped

1 bunch parsley

4 quarts filtered water

Whey (optional)

1   Peel potatoes. Place peelings, carrots and celery in a pot of water.
2   Bring to a boil, lower heat and simmer, cover for 30 minutes.
3   Allow to cool and strain into a glass container.

4 Store in refrigerator and reheat over the stove as needed. Add 1
   tbsp of whey to each cup of warm broth if desired.

ginger tea

Ginger is excellent to boost the immune system, turn off inflammation and aid in digestion. This medicinal tea is particularly helpful
for colds accompanied by coughs. Mix with honey and a bit of
lemon juice to relieve gas, bloating or menstrual cramping.

1–2 tbsp ginger
Water

1 Freshly grate or chop ginger.
2 Pour a cup of boiling water over ginger. Steep the infusion for
   10–15 minutes and then strain.

ghee-spice recipe

The ghee-spice recipe is a synergistic combination that is a simple,
yet effective way to stimulate digestion and help the body detoxify.
This is an ideal recipe to use during spring cleansing.

2 tsp ghee
1 tsp ground turmeric
1 tsp ground cumin
1 tsp ground coriander
1 tsp fennel

1 Heat ghee in a small pan.
2 Add the spices and stir to mix well, so that the aromas are
   released. Remove from heat before the spices burn.
3 Use to top seasoned cooked vegetables.

Turmeric contains the flavanoid curcumin, which is known to have anti-inflammatory properties. This wonder spice helps detoxify the liver, balance cholesterol levels, fight allergies, stimulate digestion, boost immunity and enhance the complexion. Cumin and coriander contain oils that are effective in helping to detoxify the liver and aid digestion.

When it's that time of year again—children heading back to school, after-school activities starting—the importance of the family dinner table is reinstated. In autumn, more meals are being cooked at home and this routine is the pinnacle of a successful day.

Nourishing your children is one of the most important roles you have as a parent. There is no doubt that what you feed your children impacts how they act, feel, behave and perform at school and at home. Every time you feed your kids you have the power to influence their health. The same care you put into sheltering and clothing them should also be put into feeding them properly. I imagine it won't be long before feeding children fast food and relying on processed, packaged, manufactured convenience foods to nourish them is considered a form of neglect, because it ignores their basic human needs.

It is certainly no secret that processed, packaged, manufactured and fast-food filled with trans-fats, vegetable oils, food dyes, preservatives, MSG, sugar, high fructose corn syrup, gluten and refined flours (just to name a few) contributes to, if not solely causes, the current rampant rates of obesity, Type II diabetes, cancer and ADD/ADHD among children. In fact, it has been stated that children today are going to be the sickest generation we have ever seen. Last year, I had the opportunity to lecture at several different schools. In every class, the average child was eating one litre of sugar a day. Multiply that by seven days a week and twelve months a year!

You have all seen how following your sound nutritional program has changed your symptoms, improved the way you feel, maximized your energy, alleviated brain fog and led you to better physical, mental and emotional well being. It is no different for your children. I guarantee that if you implement sound nutritional principles for your kids, you will see a marked improvement in how they function and perform at school and in their extra-curricular activities.

Following are some tips to help you supply your children with the right fuel to be successful this school year:

- Throw away all processed, packaged and manufactured foods and buy no more. I mean it!
- Eat foods that grow and subsist in nature (fruits, vegetables, fish, meat, dairy and whole gluten-free grains).
- Keep healthy food available in the fridge for when they come home, such as cut up vegetables, hummus, washed fruit, natural jerky, chicken wings, slices of real mozzarella cheese, organic yogurt, homemade trail mix, homemade soup and dried fruit.
- Give your children the gift of a healthy breakfast. Focus on eggs, protein smoothies, oatmeal, natural and pure sausages, yogurt and fresh fruit. Know that sugared cereals, fruit juices, granola bars, Pop Tarts and so on will only leave them hypoglycemic, unfocused and hyper as soon as they get to school.
- Pack a healthy lunch and snacks for your children—don't let them leave the house without fuel for the day.
- Have a healthy home-cooked dinner every night and make enough so they can take leftovers to school.
- Explain to your children why eating the foods you provide nourishes them and supports their own highest values (for example, running faster at soccer practice, better grades, more strength for dance class, more energy to walk the dog and better focus at video games). Telling your child they have to eat what you provide will not give them purpose. Teach your children how to love to eat this way by linking sound nutrition to the things that mean the most to them.

- Consider having treat day once a week—as opposed to daily treats. Daily sugar intake will negatively affect their health. You are teaching your child to appreciate occasional food pleasures as opposed to diminishing their value by taking them for granted.
- Make a list of healthy foods, meals and snacks and post it on the fridge. Involve your children in meal planning and grocery shopping.
- Transitioning your child's diet is difficult if they have been used to eating a middle-aisle grocery store diet. Put up the fight, don't give in and don't entertain their tantrums because they will eventually eat what you have prepared.

healthy snack/meal ideas for kids

Read these options to your kids and see what they would love to have or try:

- Ants on a log (celery with almond butter and raisins)
- Cut up vegetables with hummus (get different shaped vegetable cutters to make it more fun for younger children)
- Sprouted bread or rice crackers with guacamole and salsa
- Homemade trail mix (almonds, pumpkin seeds, dark chocolate chips, raisins and unsweetened shredded coconut)
- Sulfite-free dried fruit (mango, apricots, apples)
- Cut up fresh fruit with 100% nut butter and sprinkled unsweetened organic shredded coconut
- Sliced apple with nut butter and honey
- Fresh coconut chunks
- Yogurt with fresh berries and nuts
- Oven roasted chicken or turkey deli roll-ups with lettuce, cucumber, avocado and sprouts
- Natural beef, turkey or buffalo jerky

- Protein smoothies (Natural Factor's Learning Factors protein powder, berries, banana, water and coconut milk)
- Hard boiled eggs or deviled eggs
- Olives (they love putting them on their fingers!)
- Colorful salads with a creamy yogurt dressing and lots of colorful crunchy goodies
- Mozzarella cheese and veggies
- Tomato and meat sauce over spaghetti squash, rice pasta, brown rice or quinoa
- Homemade chicken and rice noodle soup
- Chicken wings and drumsticks with cut-up veggies and dip
- Pita pizzas (tomato sauce, veggies, roast chicken, natural buffalo pepperoni, pineapple, mozzarella cheese)
- Pita pocket sandwiches (cheese and cucumber, chicken and spinach, falafel, tomato and hummus)
- Small bowl of chickpeas with sea salt
- Tuna, salmon or egg salad with diced veggies and rice crackers
- Burger patties (chicken, turkey, beef, elk or bison) piled with lettuce, tomato and pickles
- Pickles and jicama

Know with certainty that you have the power to influence your child's health and performance at school with every meal and snack. Sound nutrition provides the fundamental nutrients to develop, feed and fuel your child's brain. Sound nutrition provides the nutrients to grow and develop healthy mind and spirit and to create a healthy, as opposed to a "dis-eased," body state. Sound nutrition nourishes and forms the foundation for your child to excel in whatever he/she aspires to be and do.

In autumn, routine is back in order. The kids are back in school, you're driving around the city to get to appointments and lessons, work is beckoning, the dog needs to be walked, exercise and yoga classes are starting and somewhere in between it all, a healthy nutritious dinner needs to be made. No worries my friends, there is an easy solution and one that will meet your sound nutritional needs—welcome to the world of the crock pot.

I recently set up my schedule for the fall season and found that a few nights a week my exercise and yoga classes meet later in the evening and I would not be home until 7:30 pm. It is a high value for me to eat well and eat clean whole foods every night, especially to replenish my body after a workout. The last thing I want to do is to start cooking at 7:30 pm when I'm tired and ravenous and my body is asking to be replenished and refueled. So, I bought a crock pot and discovered a newfound wonder!

Here are ten reasons why you too may want to consider making ye olde crock pot your newfound wonder.

1   It is very inexpensive (ranging from $32–$60, depending on the size of the pot).
2   It is easy to clean. At the end of the meal you have one pot and a serving spoon; you can put both in the dishwasher or easily hand wash.
3   It takes care of itself. You can leave it on all day and trust your meal will be perfectly ready for you when you get home.
4   Slow cooking is a great way to maintain nutrient content in foods. I researched this and found that nutrient loss is minimal.
5   You can have plenty of food leftover for lunches.
6   It adheres to my nutritional recommendations—you can cook lots of vegetables and high quality meats, including game and

fish. You can even cook gluten-free whole grains and legumes and make soups if you desire.

7   There are many, many free, easy and healthy crock pot recipes on the Internet. Just do a Google search. I have found recipes via the Internet that I am anxious to try (chicken and sweet potato stew, lentil soup, lamb and root vegetables, venison stew, chicken and quinoa bake). Many cookbooks are available too.

8   You don't have to be fancy—just throw some vegetables, fresh herbs and meat in the pot and call it a day (or a meal!).

9   It is convenient for the entire family, especially when schedules are different. Once the meal is cooked, keep it on the warm setting and each member of the family can have a hot meal at whatever time they come home, which also prevents reheating food in the microwave.

10 It will save you time. You still need to choose the time to buy and prepare the food, but once you have it in your home, you can either take 10–15 minutes (max) the night before and put all the food in the pot and refrigerate it overnight, or you can take the same time in the morning before you leave the house. Either way, it's little to ask for the delicious and nutritious end result.

As life starts getting hectic again, know that you don't have to compromise your health for convenience with fast food, packaged foods, dead foods, take-out or frozen dinners. Convenience and health are synthesized in the one pot wonder. No more excuses—invest in your crock pot today!

You can purchase a crock pot at various retailers including London Drugs, Home Depot, Home Outfitters, Wal-Mart, Super-store and Costco.

"Food is powerfully symbolic and really complex. Through food we express love. We bring comfort and hope. We forge new relationships and strengthen old bonds. Food reaffirms not only our humanity but the joy of being alive."[1] –Marcus Samuelsson

Many of you have experienced the healing power of foods by following my nutritional program. There is no question that food is our greatest medicine and has a tremendous effect on our physical health. But when we look at the meaning of food, there is a power that goes much deeper than the physical level. The meaning of food, unique for each of us, is rooted deeply in the mental, emotional and spiritual realms.

We create emotional memories around food. Holiday dinners, first dates, anniversaries, birthdays, nightly family suppers, the delicious smells from baking with our grandmothers, preparing meals with family members and so on have all left indelible marks on us. Food gives us the opportunity to spend time with the people who mean the most to us and in that way it becomes a very powerful identity marker.

The meaning of food is incredibly important in many religious and customary practices as well. People identify themselves and their religious beliefs with specific foods. In fact, some of my strongest impressions of food come from observing the Jewish holidays. The memories are actually symbols of celebration, belonging, tradition, family unity, love and a connection to community, knowing that thousands of other Jewish families around the world are creating the same memories. I imagine that is the same for anyone celebrating Christmas.

When people move to a different country or are away from home, they often bring foods with them or ask for care packages as a reminder of home. The connection to those specific and unique foods reminds them of what they love. The foods bring back emotions, memories, feelings and a sense of who they are. Often, all it takes is a taste of a familiar food or meal to bring back a flood of memories. It is quite profound when one bite of food can bring you back home.

Consider this story of survival. During the Holocaust as Nazis were attempting to erase identities, women kept their identities alive by sharing recipes. They referred to it as, "cooking with the mouth." In the depths of hell, women sustained their spirits by telling each other about their famous recipes. They embodied themselves in the recipes and carried the fantasy of food with them. These recipes were their connection and a symbol of love. Though the women were physically malnourished in the concentration camps, the memories and the power of what those recipes meant to them nourished their spirits and kept them alive.

The last meal is another example of how powerful the meaning of food can be. People on death row who are about to be executed make a request for one last meal. That one perfect meal can bring comfort, freedom, a reminder of home, a connection to a significant memory or family member, pleasure, power of choice, comfort, bliss, satisfaction, redemption, surrender and a connection to the soul. It is quite possible that there is a communion of body, mind and soul when that last meal is consumed.

Food is a symbol of love. Passing down recipes from generation to generation powerfully honors the people and memories we love. Cooking with family members often leaves lasting impressions and memories of love. Sharing food also speaks a profound message. When we cook with love we share a piece of ourselves with others. When we receive food in a high quality restaurant we are receiving an art and a passion from a chef who has a love and respect for food. Providing food for people affected by poverty, the Tsunami or hurricane Katrina, means providing security, hope and life—true symbols of love.

Food means so much more than just nourishment at the physical level. Food is home, love, hope, vitality, redemption and life itself. "Our attitudes, practices and rituals surrounding food are a window into our most basic beliefs about our world and ourselves."[2] Each memory we create around food will leave lasting impressions. What we eat connects us to who we are.

*"The Meaning of Food," hosted by PBS, inspired this nutrition tip. This three-part documentary series explores our relationships to food and reveals the connection food has to our identity: personal, cultural and familial. For more information visit www.PBS.org.

Using the deep rich colors and tastes of autumn foods you can create beautiful meals this season that will satisfy the soul, the senses and the stomach. The following are a few fall recipes that I offer for your enjoyment.

curried sweet potato and apple soup

2 tbsp coconut oil or butter
3 leeks, white part only, chopped
1 medium onion, chopped
2 medium carrots, chopped
2 large cloves garlic, chopped
1 tsp grated fresh ginger root
4 ½ cups vegetable or chicken broth (homemade) or organic
1 ½ lbs sweet potatoes, peeled and cut into 1–inch cubes
1 medium Granny Smith apple, cored, peeled and cubed
1 tsp curry powder
Celtic or Brittany sea salt and pepper to taste

1   Heat the oil or butter over medium heat in a soup pot. Add onion, garlic, ginger root and leeks; sauté about five minutes until onions are translucent.
2   Add remaining ingredients and stir.
3   Cover, bring to a light boil and reduce heat to low. Cook until potatoes are tender, about 1 hour.
4   Purée in batches in food processor; return to pot and heat through before serving.

cranberry wild rice bake[1]

1 cup uncooked organic wild rice

1 ½ cups water

1 tbsp olive oil

1 med organic onion, finely chopped

1 ½ cups organic chicken broth, heated

2 cloves organic garlic, minced

1 cup organic dried cranberries

1–2 tbsp black pepper

Pre-heat oven to 350°F.

2 Place rice in water and boil. Stirring occasionally. Reduce heat to low and simmer for 30 minutes. Drain.

3 Cook onion and celery in olive oil, stirring occasionally until onion is tender.

4 Mix onion, celery and rice in baking dish. Mix broth, garlic and pepper and pour over rice mixture.

5 Cover and bake 75 minutes. Stir in cranberries and bake 15–20 minutes or until liquid is absorbed.

sautéed beets[2]

3 medium organic beets, grated

½ cup organic chopped dill

2 tbsp organic butter or ghee

2 tbsp water

1 tbsp black pepper

Steam beets in water over low heat until half cooked. Add dill and butter. Steam until done.

2 Remove from heat when done to your preference. Add pepper and pinch of fresh dill.

crock-pot turkey stew[3]

2 lbs free-range turkey parts (legs, thighs, wings, breast)

1 med leek

2 stalks celery, cut into pieces

1 tsp thyme leaves

1 tsp oregano leaves

1 tsp Mrs. Dash vegetable seasoning

1 cup winter squash, peeled and cubed

1 med carrot, chopped

1 cinnamon stick

1 28-oz can tomatoes

2 cups water or chicken broth (organic)

1 Place turkey pieces, skin-side down in crock-pot set on high, and start to sauté to release fat. Turn turkey pieces and add leeks and celery. Sprinkle on thyme, oregano and vegetable seasoning, and sauté until leeks become translucent.

2 Add squash, carrots, cinnamon stick, tomatoes and broth, and simmer covered, for 2–3 hours on medium or up to 6–8 hours on lowest setting.

red velvet soup

1 cup red lentils, soaked 4–8 hours

1 tbsp butter

1 large onion, chopped

2 large carrots, chopped

2 beets, peel ends and chop

3 bay leaves

6 cups water or vegetable broth

1 tbsp miso

1 tsp Celtic or Brittany sea salt

Parsley, finely chopped

1 Drain and rinse the lentils.
2 Heat butter in soup pot and sauté onion for 5 minutes, stirring frequently with a wooden spoon.
3 Add lentils, water or broth, carrots, beets and bay leaves; bring slowly to boil. Lower heat and simmer covered for 1 hour until lentils and vegetables are very soft.
4 Remove bay leaves and discard. Purée vegetables in food processor or blender.
5 Dissolve miso in ½ cup water and add to soup. (If soup is too thick, add more water.)
6 Heat soup gently, 5 to 10 minutes.
7 Garnish with chopped parsley and serve.

"Beans, beans, the magical fruit,
The more you eat them, the more you toot,
The more you toot, the better you feel,
So eat your beans at every meal."

I'm not sure where that lyrical adage originated but it is one I'm sure many of you remember chanting during childhood when beans were served for dinner (or maybe that was just in my family?). Though of course I don't recommend beans at every meal, they certainly are a magical food.

Legumes are the edible seeds of leguminous plants, which abound in many more varieties than any other vegetable (peas, broad beans, haricot beans, lentils and so on). Legumen (edible seeds which form in pods) is derived from the Latin verb lego, which means to gather, collect, to choose, select or to take. According to *History of Food* by Maguelonne Toussaint-Samat, "in ancient times when men were out hunting women used their feminine wisdom to gather and collect nutritious plants."[1]

Leguminous vegetables are very nutritious because of the starch, protein and high mineral profile they contain. One cup of beans can provide 6–7 grams of fibre, nutrients such as potassium, iron and thiamine, 12 grams of complex carbohydrates and 17 grams of protein. Legumes are a fantastic source of protein for vegetarians as well as for meat-lovers who want a lighter meal from time to time. They have been described as "the poor man's meat."

It is important to note that legumes are not a complete protein, meaning they do not have the eight amino acids necessary to make a true protein source such as meat, fish and eggs. So when you eat legumes combine them with nuts, seeds or whole grains, because those foods have the missing amino acids which when consumed together with legumes then make a perfect protein.

Cooking beans from scratch certainly does not make for the most time-efficient meal (unless you have a crock pot—see Tip 67) so experiment on the weekends or when you have more time. During the week, canned organic beans can be used and are recommended as part of your regular nutritional intake. They are a quick and easy protein addition to salads. Purchase a variety of natural beans (garbanzo, black-eyed, pinto, adzuki, kidney, lentils, mung, lima and so on) and rinse them well before using to wash away all starchy by-products. Even though they are a canned food, these beans do maintain their high fibre and nutrient content. Buy organic brands, which are free of preservatives and other harmful ingredients. Note that I am recommending canned organic beans. This does not include canned processed products like baked beans or pork and beans, which are full of sugar, sodium, MSG, hydrogenated oils and high fructose corn syrup.

For some people, beans are difficult to digest. Because they have low agni (digestive fire) vata types typically do well only with lentils, mung beans and chickpeas and are not able to break down bigger beans such as kidney or lima beans. Pitta types have lots of agni so they can usually tolerate beans much better than vata types. Kapha types also do well with legumes as long as they use stimulating spices and herbs to aid in digestion, as listed below. It is my experience that when cooked properly legumes are actually digestive friendly but using digestive enzymes at a meal with beans is also beneficial.

In *Transition to Vegetarianism,* Dr. Rudolph Ballentine recommends the following tips to make beans less gassy:

- Generally smaller beans are more digestible (e.g., Mung beans, black beans, adzuki, pinto beans, compared with kidney or lima beans).

- Soak beans overnight, and then discard the soaking water. This eliminates some gas-forming substances and brings beans out of dormancy.
- Rinse beans well and continue to discard water until it runs clear. Then refill pot with fresh water.
- Cook beans until well done—beans should be soft enough to mash between fingers.
- If water needs to be added during cooking, it should be boiling hot.
- Season beans with spices that stimulate digestion such as turmeric, cumin, coriander, ginger, black mustard seeds, cardamom, cloves and black pepper. Herbs such as thyme, sage and marjoram can also be used. Onions, seaweeds and garlic also help stimulate digestion.
- Add sea salt and oil to cooking water.
- Near the end of cooking add acid seasonings such as tomato, vinegar or lemon juice and allow simmering for 10–15 minutes more.
- Cook with enough water to make a dilute dish and serve in small quantities with whole gluten-free grains or nuts and seeds and leafy green vegetables.[2]

The following is one of my favorite bean recipes that is perfect for the fall and winter season. Don't be deterred by the long list of ingredients, they are mostly herbs and spices. It is quick to prepare and tastes even better the next day. Cocoa is the secret ingredient it deepens the color and rounds out the flavor.

easy vegetarian chili[3]

1 tbsp olive oil

2 onions, chopped

2 green and/or red peppers, chopped

3 cloves garlic, crushed

2 cups mushrooms, sliced

2 cups cooked or canned red kidney beans

2 cups cooked or canned chickpeas

1 ½ cups bulgar or couscous rinsed (If you are sensitive to wheat use 1 cup quinoa or millet. If using millet, cook on medium heat for 5 minutes to brown, before adding to recipe.)

28-oz can tomatoes or 6 fresh tomatoes, chopped

1 cup bottled salsa, mild or medium

1 ½ cup water

1 tsp salt

1 tbsp chili powder

1 tsp dried basil

1 ½ tsp each pepper, oregano, cumin

1 ½ tsp cayenne

1 tbsp unsweetened cocoa powder

1 tsp sugar (optional)

1 Heat oil in large pot.
2 Sauté onions, peppers and garlic for 5 minutes on medium heat. Add mushrooms and sauté 4–5 minutes more. Add remaining ingredients.
3 Bring to a boil and simmer covered for 25 minutes, stirring occasionally.

Yields 10 servings. Freezes and reheats well.

creating the sacred table

"We acknowledge the gift of food from the Divine and ask that by eating we support our highest purpose and intention—that is to know ourselves and all the universe as an expression of divine consciousness." –interpretation from the *Bhagavad Gita* in Sanskrit

I trust that you are all adopting your nutritional recommendations as a lifestyle. My hope is that you have made your nutrition a higher priority, you have linked it to your highest values, you spend time cooking, shopping, preparing snacks and meals for work, have eliminated all processed, packaged, manufactured foods, are focusing only on live, natural whole foods, have eliminated the foods that trigger your symptoms and consume only the foods you know will create wellness in your body.

The next step stems from asking the question, "Are you actually eating when you eat?" Are you fully present, grateful and connected to what you are putting into your body? In Tip 35, I wrote, "Nutrition is the science, but nourishment is the soul, and merging these two truths is the key to helping you achieve optimum wellness." Most of us fail to eat when we actually eat, so this tip invites you to consider the importance of connecting with your food and creating a sacred table.

Nourishing your body can be one of the most pleasing, satisfying, health-promoting and enjoyable experiences. We have the opportunity to gift ourselves this pleasure with every meal, yet often we deny ourselves this gift. Sometimes, the cause is the choice called "no time". Sometimes, the cause is ignorance— minimal awareness of the significance to health and wellness of nourishing the body versus eating the food. Eating with awareness is one critical element of nutritional mastery. The more relaxed, grateful, aware and connected you are the more nourishment you receive from your food.

As you journey to optimal wellness, consider making the following practices a part of your nutritional lifestyle:

- Create a beautiful plate with lots of colors and vitality. The
  more pleasing your plate looks the more pleasure you will
  receive from your food.
- Eat slowly. Chew every bite, relish in the flavors, aroma and
  textures of the foods. Stimulating the senses can release
  mood-elevating hormones, so allow your meal to be the
  pick-me-up you need.
- Sit and enjoy your meal. Avoid getting up from the table
  10–15 times. If you have young children, consider eating
  before or after them so you can actually enjoy and taste
  your meal.
- Create a mantra and chant it inwardly while you eat, such
  as "I know this food will bring me good health and nourish
  my body." The more you believe in the power of food and tell
  your body it will support your healing and wellness goals, the
  more it will work for you.
- Digest your food for a few minutes after a meal. Avoid getting
  up to clear the dishes while chewing your last bite. There is
  nothing more important in those few moments than to give
  your body the time to assimilate the nutrients.
- Tap into how you feel after every meal. Are you satisfied,
  satiated, and free of cravings and do you have a sense of
  mental, emotional and physical well being? If you experience
  these things then you know your meal was right for you.

Eating is not merely a physical act. There is an incredible spiritual
component to food and when you tap into that you receive the
most out of your nutrition. That is why I recommend that you create

a sacred table. If your lifestyle doesn't permit you to do it at every meal, at least once a day create a sacred eating place.

the recipe to create your sacred table

1 nice tablecloth or colorful sari on your table

2 candles

1 CD you love and that relaxes you

1 bunch fresh flowers weekly to put in the middle of the table

1 phone off the hook

1 mantra to chant inwardly while eating

Yourself and/or family and friends

10 deep belly breaths before and after you eat

The intention to have a nice relaxed meal, conversation, or time with yourself

1 colorful plate of food that you know will nourish your body and help you achieve your health goals

So, it's not just about the food. It's how we accept, acknowledge and receive our food that can take our nutrition potential that much further. Create your sacred table and when you eat, truly eat with purpose, intention and love and I guarantee you will receive more out of your food than you ever thought possible.

Dr. Andrew Weil states, "By definition, diets are regimens that eventually end." Sound nutrition, on the other hand, is an infinite journey of growth that can only come from challenges and successes along the way.

Many of you have heard me say that perfection is over-rated. If you expect to be perfect with your nutrition 100% of the time, I guarantee you will set yourself up for failure. Consider how everything else in your life operates. There will be days you are kind toward your family and days you are a tyrant. There will be weeks when your business is busy and weeks when it slows down. You may have a month when you are really social followed by a month of being with yourself. There will be days when you feel gratitude for all that is as it is and days when you will want to change your reality. You'll have months when your finances are in order and months when there never seems to be enough money. There will be times when you read nightly and nights where you can't be bothered to pick up a book.

In every area of your life you constantly oscillate between action and inaction and challenges and successes, but you'll never find yourself throwing the towel in on any of the areas mentioned above. View your nutritional lifestyle the same way. Just as with everything else in your life, your nutrition will oscillate between good and bad days, challenges and successes, a few pounds gained and a few lost, meals at the sacred table and meals skipped or rushed, a clean week and a week with poorer quality food. The key is not to give up or get attached to one side—or believe you should only have one side. Know that it is completely natural to constantly wave between the two sides.

Your life is an infinite journey and so your nutritional lifestyle is one as well. When you give up and finite the possibility of growth (which can only come from challenges and successes) you have put yourself already on yet another diet.

My nutritional program is not designed to be a diet. Clients come in for adjustments, for more variety when they are feeling bored and stagnant, for support when they are feeling challenged. Clients come in to transition their foods seasonally, to work on emotional triggers, to say, "Something doesn't feel right. I want to try something new," to reintroduce and retest foods after eliminations, to learn to tap into how foods make them feel after eating the ones they know they need to avoid. Clients come in for motivation when feeling stuck, to be held accountable to meet goals, to continue to work on linking nutrition to highest values, and to learn more about Ayurveda, metabolic typing and other important areas of nutrition. These are the clients who are truly on the infinite journey.

Clients who tossed the sound nutrition program in the pile with all the other diet books finite their own possibility of growth. Somehow these are the people who believe or expect that their nutritional programs should be only one-sided—meaning easy without hard, success without challenges, results without adjustments.

Diet-consciousness seems to expect perfection, and people who "fail" to reach that finite expectation feel that they have no willpower or that they are weak. Nutrition-consciousness includes knowing that two sides exist always; that your successes and triumphs cannot come without challenge and effort. Isn't that true for all areas of your life? When the going gets tough with your business, family, friends or finances you don't give up, so why do you feel your nutritional lifestyles are any different?

Along the path to optimum wellness through sound nutrition you will experience intermittent moments of growth. You might have a tear in your eye when you reach your first weight loss goal, feel grateful for your first day in years without pain, beam with delight for the newfound energy you haven't felt since you were young, experience inner peace when you created and nourished yourself at your sacred table. Perhaps you know a moment of great clarity when you overcome your emotional trigger that led you to overeating; or you open your heart to yourself and your family when you create and cook a vibrant, healthy, colorful meal; and you will have a moment of deep satisfaction with yourself for stopping and taking the time to make a better food choice. Each of these moments makes up your lighted moments—your moments of growth. Every time you reach that lighted moment you have moved another step on your infinite journey. Those moments of growth last for a moment, though, as growth is not finite. When that moment is over, you can be assured you will meet the next challenge you will need to overcome to take you to your next intermittent moment of light.

It is important to avoid getting stuck in the moments of success and have an expectation that the rest of your nutritional lifestyle should stay like that. It is not possible. Every new success will bring a new challenge and every challenge will bring new success. Your growth is dependent on both. You have infinite potential for growth on your journey to optimum wellness through sound nutrition, so don't limit what is possible for yourself. Welcome both sides, knowing that both exist so you can grow.

In your nutritional recommendations, I always emphasize that meat, eggs and dairy should be organic, grass fed and free-range for several reasons: to avoid second generation carbohydrates which increase saturated fat, to reduce the intake of omega-6 fats which can trigger silent inflammation, and to avoid harmful hormones and antibiotics. For those who have yet to adopt this recommendation, this nutrition tip may change your mind. For those who follow this recommendation—after reading this article, you will be grateful that you have made that leap of faith.

The other night, I watched a very disturbing yet eye-opening documentary called "Frankensteer" on CBC's "The Passionate Eye." It reinforced what I already knew: organic meat, especially beef, is important to your health.

consider the following

Biologically speaking, cows always were meant to eat grass. We started to feed them grain and corn to fatten them up for human consumption. As you might already know from our teaching sessions, grain-fed cattle has 50% saturated fat whereas grass-fed cows only have 10% saturated fat. It is no coincidence that this is the ratio we're also finding in humans. Metabolically and genetically, just like cattle, we were not meant to fuel on grains. The more grain we eat, the fatter and sicker we get. One of the major cattle farmers in Southern Alberta said that you have to introduce this crop to cows very slowly as their stomachs do not recognize nor know how to break it down. They can end up getting lactic acidosis, which is fatal.

Grain and corn also happen to be cheap, so if one of the major goals of the cattle industry is to lower the cost of production, overriding nature might not be a significant deterrent. Consider also that grain-fed cattle intended for slaughter spend their lives in stressful feedlots. Contrast that with free range cattle that spend their first six to eight months feeding on grass.

Hormones and antibiotics are injected into commercial cattle. You might be shocked to know that 50% of the total tonnage of antibiotics used in Canada ends up in livestock. While all of Europe has banned the use of antibiotics and hormones in cattle because science showed that they are harmful to humans (especially to children and pregnant mothers), Canada and the U.S. continue to still use them. Dr. Shiv Chopra, a veterinary scientist with Health Canada, reported that Estradiol (the growth hormone of choice for cattle), shrinks their thymus glands (regulator of immunity), enlarges the uterus and is known to cause cancer in humans, especially breast cancer. He was challenged—not about his findings, but for reporting them publicly.

When cattle producers and government agencies decided they wanted to fatten the cattle up even more than they already had, they decided to use protein to do so. Animal by-product and remains as feed was the next brilliant idea. As a result, BSE/Mad Cow Disease arrived. By the way, if you think that all cattle are being tested for BSE, know that they are not. One of the farmers on the documentary said that less than 2% of all cows that get slaughtered are tested for BSE. Another startling piece of news revealed by the documentary is that feedlots are feeding slaughtered cows' blood to calves because there is no "definitive science" that has proven that it causes BSE.

The Veterinarian Specialists and the Canadian Heath Coalition have said that you need to treat your meat as toxic material, being especially cautions of the deadly E. coli bacteria that results from feeding animal remains to animals. There is talk now about radiating beef to kill this E. Coli strain. For us humans, the more radiation we are exposed to, the higher the incidence of cancer we find.

Know that it is so important that you eat organic, grass-fed, free-range beef. I know it is considerably more expensive, but given its value for your life, does that really matter? The farmers in the documentary believe that the producer will produce what the consumer demands. The more we become aware of what is truly happening in the cattle industry, the more demand there will be for farmers to change their ways. It is possible to develop safe and clean markets, it would cost more per steer, but for the betterment of our health and for the health of the cattle, I'd say it is worth it.

It is time to support the certified organic farms in Alberta or in your area that raise beef naturally and healthily. They use no sprays or chemical fertilizers, the cows have space to roam, the cattle feed on grass, they are not injected with hormones, antibiotics or force-fed animal by-product. These farmers produce animals that are in as natural an environment as possible. When stressing over the cost of organic beef, know that you are supporting yourself and people who care about animals and health. You are supporting the people who are against the use of cancer-causing hormones. You are supporting people who take care of the environment and believe that cows should be treated and raised naturally. You are supporting people who have humbled themselves to Mother Nature and haven't tried to change Her ways.

It's sad but true. Man has created Frankensteer—"an antibiotic-dependant, hormone-laced, potential carrier of toxic bacteria."[1] You have the choice and now the knowledge. Don't feed the system that's feeding you toxic food. Support the system that supports your health.

Oh December! The month of indulgence! Whether it's indulging in food, shopping, socializing, drinking, partying or holidaying, everything about it is big and expansive.

In the act of indulgence it almost seems as if we lose a bit of our true selves or become disconnected from who we really are. As you were forcing that last big meal in your gut knowing you were stuffed from the five previous large meals you had, were you truly connected to your self? As your credit card seemed to leave your wallet more than you wanted it to, were you truly making conscious decisions? When you continued to go out and socialize even though you knew you were exhausted and just wanted to stay home, did you ever feel as though you weren't really in your body?

It's hard to avoid the holiday indulgences. But January is a perfect time to get back in touch with ourselves and what it is that we most value. I think we are all grateful when the holiday season is over and we can get back to our routines, eating well, exercising and refocusing our attention at work. But no need to feel guilty about the month of indulgence because we all do it, every year, and perhaps we need to go big before we go home.

As Elson Haas writes in *Staying Healthy with the Seasons,*

> Winter is a more inward and sensitive time. It is a time to be deeper within yourself, seeking replenishment, resting, reflecting and being more aware of your senses. It is the time to hibernate at home, get plenty of rest, good nutrition, relaxation and sleep.[1]

So, leave the holidays behind as a memory and know that now is the time and season to come back home—to yourself. Get back into your routines, back to the gym, back to making soups and meals that will warm you on a cool winter night, back to seeing me for a nutrition follow up, back to meditating, doing yoga, back to staying at home and relaxing on your sofa at night and back to whatever hobby, activity or project that makes you connected to you (such as knitting, playing guitar, piano, being in the mountains, working on the house or reading).

Welcome home everybody…

I would like to share with you my life mission statement:

> I have dedicated my life to inspiring, educating and motivating
> people to realize the significant impact sound nutrition has on
> achieving optimum wellness.

> The 7 Steps to Sound Nutrition™ is the most comprehensive
> approach to nutrition. It combines scientific, holistic, Eastern
> and Western insights including nutritional biochemistry, meta-
> bolic typing, Ayurvedic nutrition, connecting the mind and body
> through soulful nourishment, and seasonal eating. Each step
> of the program provides tools and a deep understanding of
> how our physical, mental, emotional and spiritual well being
> is greatly influenced by the foods we eat and the relationship
> these foods have with the health of our unique bodies. My cli-
> ents have the realization that their wellness is a result of their
> dedication to their nutritional journeys. This awareness provides
> them with a foundation to create and live the lives they desire
> and love.

> By actualizing my vocational mission, I will have the means to
> live the life that I desire—my own journey of growth, fulfillment
> and mastery in all of the areas of my life. An infinite journey
> from quantum to quantum that will provide me with the inspira-
> tion, education and motivation to live according to my values,
> to love who I am, to see the perfection in all that surrounds me
> and to take this wisdom and live my life in moments of love,
> light and gratitude.

One of my goals as your Nutritional Consulting Practitioner is to create an awareness of your nutritional choices and help you to make a shift in your consciousness. It is not enough to take the customized nutritional program I create for you in Step Two and try it for a short period of time. It does not serve you to follow your program only until your symptoms have improved, only to revert back to old patterns. It is life limiting to view nutrition simply as a means to satiate physical hunger or feed an emotional misperception. Your nutritional program is designed to enhance your entire being—body, mind and spirit/soul. Your sound nutrition is your foundation for living. It provides you with the energy, chi, prana and life force to help you achieve your aspirations in life. It fuels you to fulfill your mission and purpose in life.

When I recommend that you eat the foods that grow and subsist in nature and avoid all processed, packaged, and manufactured foods, I do so because it serves your life, enabling you to resonate with greater energy and higher frequency. You resonate with the level of energy of the foods you eat. If you are eating live, whole food, you are emitting magnetic, vibrant energy. If you are eating foods from cans, bottles, foods that sit on store shelves for months at a time, have prizes in the boxes, are created in a factory, etc. you are eating dead food and you are fueling on dead energy.

I recommend that you shop at the health food stores and farmer's markets. By shopping there, you connect to a greater community of people who care about their health and environment, and have a great respect for the power of foods. As one owner of a farmer's market states,

> Magically and inevitably, the farmers and their food create a
> human space that links us back to the most ancient centers of
> civilization as well as to the present cycles of nature.[1]

This, too, promotes wellness.

When I recommend high-quality organic food, it is so that you can have access to the magnificence of the greatest gifts from Mother Nature. These whole living foods, free of harmful chemicals and toxins, have a more nourishing and vitalizing effect on both body and mind. The food might be more costly but consider its value.

> When food is cheap, we tend to treat it carelessly and wastefully. But when it's dear, when it costs what it's actually worth, we tend to pay closer attention to it. In this sense, good food can sharply focus our world.[2]

When I recommend that you take and make the time to shop, prepare and cook meals it is so you move toward a beautiful relationship with your food. To create a colorful, fresh, vibrant plate of food is an art and a gift to yourself and others with whom you choose to share it. It is an opportunity to slow down, connect, and be in touch with nature, family, friends and your self. Cooking like this nourishes you daily.

When I recommend that you transition your diet with the seasons, it is so you are in sync with nature's cycles and know the foods grown in specific seasons are there to support our bodies for specific reasons at those given times. When you are not in touch with those cycles, vitality diminishes and you become less aware of the subtleties that surround you.

When I recommend that you tap into how you are feeling after you eat certain foods it is so you can attune to your body's own innate wisdom. When you listen to your "gut" or your inner voice, you are trusting your God-given intuition. When you are disconnected to those important messages you are unconscious.

When I recommend that you work on Step Five to overcome emotional blocks and barriers around your food, it is so you can see that addictions, habits and poor nutritional choices are merely cover-ups for unconscious thought patterns. Once you are aware of the fact of those thought patterns, you can then become more conscious to the inner work that precedes optimum wellness. Your emotional body provides you the opportunity to go inward so you can move forward on your journey to wellness.

When I recommend you create variety in your diet it is so you realize a kaleidoscope of tastes, colors, textures and scents exist that will stimulate your senses. Eating for sight, smell, touch and sound will elevate your being and allow you to become spiritually connected to your food.

When I recommend that you eat with gratitude and tell your body that the food you are about to receive will help move you toward optimum wellness, it is so you are connecting to a greater power. Gratitude means "state of grace," and giving thanks to a force beyond yourself is a healing act.

When I recommend that you believe in the power of foods it is so you can surrender to nature's perfection. Our greatest medicine is our food. Those of you who are my clients and to those who have worked to optimize your nutrition all have seen that the slightest eliminations, additions and adjustments to your diet can make a significant difference in how you feel physically, mentally, emotionally and spiritually. Stay present to this power.

When I recommend that you eat clean food it is so you will enjoy a clear mind, pure body and acute awareness—all of which are necessary to tap into your higher mind and true self.

When I recommend that you cook and eat with love it is so you know… there simply is no other way to nourish.

My greatest desire is for you to maintain your nutritional lifestyle indefinitely. I hope that you do so not because you have to or need to, but because you choose to and love to—because you have experienced the power of the truths I have written. "Food is indeed universal consciousness—and it alters our individual consciousness."[3] Once you experience that for yourself, the unhealthy eating habits you have been trying so hard to overcome will vanish and sound nutrition will become your reality. That, my friends, is when you will have mastered your nutrition.

tip 2

1 Daniel, Dr. Kaayla. *The Whole Soy Story: The Dark Side of America's Favorite Health Food.* New Trends Publishing. 2005.
2 www.mercola.com

tip 3

1 Health Canada. "Nutrient Value of Some Common Foods." 1999.
2 Canadian Bison Association. *Smoke Signals.* Manitoba. 2004.

tip 5

1 Toussaint-Samat, Maguelonne. Translated by Anthea Bell. *History of Food.* Blackwell Publishers Ltd: Massachussets. 2001.
2 Edwards, Bonnie. *America's Favorite Drug: Coffee and Your Health.* Odonian Press. 1992.

tip 6

1 Pitchford, Paul. *Healing with Whole Foods.* 3rd ed. North Atlantic Books: California. 2002.

tip 8

1 Rowland, David. *The Nutritional Bypass: Reverse Atherosclerosis without Surgery.* Rowland Publications: Ontario. 1995.
2 Fallon, Sally. *Nourishing Traditions.* New Trends Publishing: Washington. 2001.
3 Ravnskov, Uffe, MD, PhD. *The Cholesterol Myths: Exposing the Fallacy that Saturated Fat and Cholesterol cause Heart Disease.* New Trends Publishing: Washington. 2000.
4 Null, Gary, PhD. *The Complete Encyclopedia of Natural Healing.* Bottom Line Books. 2004.
5 Fallon, Sally. *Nourishing Traditions.* New Trends Publishing: Washington. 2001.

tip 9

1 Rogers, Sherry A. *Pain Free in 6 Weeks.* Prestige Pubs. 2001.

tip 10

1 www.mercola.com
2 Colgan, Dr. Michael. *Optimum Sports Nutrition.* Advanced Research Press: New York. 1993.
3 www.mercola.com
4 Ibid.
5 Ibid.

tip 11

1 Douillard, John. *The 3-Season Diet.* Three Rivers Press: New York. 2000.

tip 12

1 Cordain, Dr. Loren. *The Paleolithic Diet.* John Wiley and Sons Inc: New Jersey. 2000.
2 Spreen, Dr. Allan. "Carbohydrates: The Real Truth About Carbohydrates." Interview. 2003.
3 Embry, Ashton. "Nutritional Strategies for Controlling MS." *Direct-MS.* 1994.

tip 13

1 www.mercola.com

tip 16

1 www.mercola.com
2 Ibid.

tip 18

1 www.drdemartini.com

tip 19

1 Pitchford, Paul. *Healing with Whole Foods.* 3rd ed. North Atlantic Books: California. 2002.
2 Ballentine, Dr. Rudolph. *Radical Healing.* Three Rivers Press: New York. 1999.
3 Ibid.
4 Ballentine, Dr. Rudolph. *Diet & Nutrition; A Holistic Approach.* Himalayan International Institute: Pennsylvania. 1987.

tip 20

1 Douillard, John. *The 3-Season Diet.* Three Rivers Press: New York. 2000.

tip 21

1 Mercola, Dr. Joseph. *Dr. Mercola's Total Health Cookbook and Program.* Mercola.com: Shaumburg, IL. 2003.

tip 22

1 Douillard, John. *The 3-Season Diet.* Three Rivers Press: New York. 2000.

tip 23

1 Gilletz, Norene. *Meal Leani Yumm.* ISBN: 0-9697972-2-2
2 *Homemakers.* May 1998.
3 Nutrition Action Healthletter. November 2003.
4 Ibid.

tip 24

1 Mercola, Dr. Joseph. *Dr. Mercola's Total Health Cookbook and Program.* Mercola.com: Shaumburg, IL. 2003.
2 Ibid.

tip 25

1 Jensen, Bernard. *The Chemistry of Man.* Bernard Jensen:
   CA. 1983.
2 Ibid.
3 Fallon, Sally. *Nourishing Traditions.* New Trends Publishing:
   Washington. 2001.

tip 31

1 Gilletz, Norene. *Meal Leani Yumm.* ISBN: 0-9697972-2-2

tip 33

1 Mayhew, Debra. *The Soup Bible.* Anness Publishing Ltd.:
   London. 2002.
2 Ibid.
3 Ibid.
4 Ibid.

tip 35

1 David, Mark. "Eating from the Tree: Nutrition Lessons for the
   Scientific Soul." *Alternative Therapies.* Nov/Dec 2004. Vol. 10,
   No. 6.
2 Ibid.
3 Ibid.
4 Ibid.

tip 37

1 Perricone, Nicholas. *The Perricone Promise.* Warner Books: New
   York. 2004.
2 Ibid.

tip 38

1 Mercola, Dr. Joseph. *Dr. Mercola's Total Health Cookbook and
   Program.* Mercola.com: Shaumburg, IL. 2003.

tip 39

1 www.mercola.com

tip 40

1 Mercola, Dr. Joseph. *Dr. Mercola's Total Health Cookbook and Program.* Mercola.com: Shaumburg, IL. 2003.
2 Rosedale, Ron. "Insulin and Its Metabolic Effects." Interview. August 1999.
3 Mercola, Dr. Joseph. *Dr. Mercola's Total Health Cookbook and Program.* Mercola.com: Shaumburg, IL. 2003.
4 Ibid.

tip 41

1 *Organic Lifestyles.* Vol. 1, Issue 3.

tip 44

1 Haas, Elson. *Staying Healthy With the Seasons.* Celestial Arts: Toronto. 2003.

tip 47

1 Mercola, Dr. Joseph. *Dr. Mercola's Total Health Cookbook and Program.* Mercola.com: Shaumburg, IL. 2003.
2 Ibid.

tip 49

1 Erasmus, Udo. *Fats that Heal, Fats that Kill.* Alive Books: Canada.1993.
2 www.mercola.com
3 *The Complete Guide to Natural Healing.* International Masters Publishing Inc.

tip 53

1 Wallace, Dr. Jeanne. "General Recommendations for a Healthy Diet." (Publishing information not found).
2 Ibid.

tip 58

1 Douillard, John. *The 3-Season Diet.* Three Rivers Press: New York. 2000.

tip 60

1 Colgan, Dr. Michael. *Optimum Sports Nutrition.* Advanced Research Press: New York. 1993.

tip 61

1 Rountree, Robert. "Brassica Vegetables and Glucosinolates: Their Role in Detoxification and Health." Bouldar Wellcare, 2005.

tip 63

1 Wolcott, William and Trish Fahey. *The Metabolic Typing Diet.* Broadway Books: New York. 2000.
2 Ibid.

tip 65

1 Fallon, Sally. *Nourishing Traditions.* New Trends Publishing: Washington. 2001.
2 Pitchford, Paul. *Healing with Whole Foods.* 3rd ed. North Atlantic Books: California. 2002.
3 Fallon, Sally. *Nourishing Traditions.* New Trends Publishing: Washington. 2001.

tip 68

1 www.pbs.org. "The Meaning of Food." (Documentary) 2005.
2 Ibid.

tip 69

1 Harrison, Katrina & Carol Howden. *Ancient Wisdom In Modern Menu.* Canada: 2005.
2 Ibid.
3 Mercola, Dr. Joseph. *Dr. Mercola's Total Health Cookbook and Program.* Mercola.com: Shaumburg, IL. 2003.

tip 70

1 Toussaint-Samat, Maguelonne. Translated by Anthea Bell. *History of Food.* Blackwell Publishers Ltd: Massachussets. 2001.
2 Ballentine, Rudolph. *Transition to Vegetarianism.* The Himalayan Institute Press: Pennsylvania. 1999.
3 Gilletz, Norene. *Meal Leani Yumm.* ISBN: 0-9697972-2-2

tip 73

1 CBC—"Frankensteer." (Documentary) 2005.

tip 74

1 Haas, Elson. *Staying Healthy With the Seasons.* Celestial Arts: Toronto. 2003.

tip 75

1 Madison, Deborah. "Local Markets: Biodiversity you can Taste." *Yoga International.* Issue no. 85. September 2005.
2 Ibid.
3 Ibid.

>what am i holding on to? (Tip 55)

my commitment list for creating a sound nutritional lifestyle

my commitment list for creating a sound
nutritional lifestyle (cont'd)

reflections

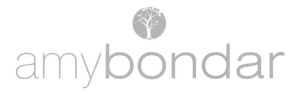

amybondar

Amy Bondar (BSW, MSc, NCP) has dedicated her life to inspiring, educating and motivating people to realize the significant impact sound nutrition has on achieving optimum wellness.

She earned a Masters of Applied Science in Nutrition, building on her degree in Clinical Social Work. Amy has created and developed the 7 Steps to Sound Nutrition™ program—possibly North America's most all-encompassing approach to nutrition. It combines scientific, holistic, Eastern and Western insights to provide you with a customized nutritional road map that enables you to actualize your health goals according to your body's unique needs.

It is Amy's commitment, process and personal journey to stay at the forefront of the latest nutritional information and research so she can ensure the utmost certainty and care when creating your customized nutritional program. Amy's knowledge and passion is contagious. She encourages and invites you to work with her as you journey toward optimum wellness through sound nutrition.

to continue the journey, visit www.amybondar.com